Michael Lynagh won 72 Test caps and retired from international rugby in 1995 as the world record points scorer with 911, a total which remains an Australian record. An inspirational playmaker, Lynagh, who also won 100 caps for Queensland, made his Test debut in 1984 and was part of Australia's Grand Slam-winning team later that year. He was vice-captain of Australia's World Cup-winning side in 1991 and, after captaining Australia to the quarter-finals of the 1995 World Cup, he retired from international rugby and joined Saracens in the UK at the start of the professional era.

BLINDSIDED

MICHAEL LYNAGH

with Mark Eglinton

HarperSport
An Imprint of HarperCollinsPublishers

HarperSport
An imprint of HarperCollins*Publishers*
1 London Bridge Street
London SE1 9GF

www.harpercollins.co.uk

First published in Australia by
HarperCollins*Publishers* Australia Pty Limited 2015
First published in the UK by HarperCollins*Publishers* 2015

10 9 8 7 6 5 4 3 2 1

Cover design by HarperCollins Design Studio
Typeset in Sabon LT by Kirby Jones

A catalogue record of this book is
available from the British Library

HB ISBN 978-0-00-756874-1
TPB ISBN 978-0-00-814439-5

Printed and bound in Great Britain by
Clays Ltd, St Ives plc

MIX
Paper from
responsible sources
FSC **FSC C007454**
www.fsc.org

FSC is a non-profit international organisation established to promote
the responsible management of the world's forests. Products carrying the
FSC label are independently certified to assure consumers that they come
from forests that are managed to meet the social, economic and
ecological needs of present and future generations,
and other controlled sources.

Find out more about HarperCollins and the environment at
www.harpercollins.co.uk/green

CONTENTS

FOREWORD
by Alan Jones

IN 1984, I HAD inherited the Wallabies coaching job in fairly difficult and controversial circumstances. The Wallabies, over time, had rarely achieved according to their potential. I was encouraged by players to apply for the coaching job and I was successful.

I can say what I've never said before, that I was genuinely excited by the talent at my disposal. Amongst that talent was a remarkable twenty year old from Queensland, Michael Lynagh. Rugby was fortunate that he was still within our ranks. He was a gifted schoolboy cricketer; but I suspect he would have been good at anything that remotely resembled a ball sport. As a recreational golfer, he was as good as anybody.

I soon learnt on becoming coach that we had in front of us, in 1984, a very difficult tour of Britain, subsequently to be known as the Grand Slam Tour. But before that, we had the domestic season to deal with and the mighty All Blacks were touring Australia.

We won the first Test magnificently in Sydney, in what could only be described as a rugby boilover. But in something of a kicking duel, where we were almost embarrassingly without a kicker in Brisbane, we lost in a whistle-blowing affair by one point.

Already, the '84 Wallabies had served notice to the rest of the world. The showdown third Test was to be in Sydney. In the lead-up to Sydney, Queensland, with Michael playing, had been hammered by the All Blacks. I sensed that Michael Lynagh was the secret weapon that we needed for Sydney, a brilliant and gifted goal-kicker.

I pulled him aside after the Queensland vs. All Blacks game into an empty dressing room. He had never played in a run-on side for Australia. After all, he was only twenty. I told him that we didn't know one another very well, but I wanted him for Sydney as the goal-kicker. I felt it would be a penalty showdown. Typically Michael Lynagh, he was worried about who he would be replacing, and he asked me who. I gently suggested that was my worry—I just wanted him to play. He told me that he'd never played on the Sydney Cricket Ground and he thought he might let me down.

In the conversation that ensued, I gained a telling insight into this remarkable Australian. He was gifted, yes. He was modest beyond dimension. I told him I didn't want anyone playing if they were unhappy about the assignment I was asking of them. We left the meeting with the understanding that he wouldn't be picked. I chose to accommodate his concerns ahead of the urgent needs of Australian rugby.

We went to Sydney and in the virtual penalty shoot-out with a whistle-happy Northern Hemisphere referee, we lost a critical, indeed historic, Test by one point. But in a way, the dye had been cast. I knew Michael would be central to changing the fortunes of Australian rugby.

And he was.

He was always a worrier. Early on, on that Grand Slam tour, he had a whinge to me about the praise I was giving at training to Mark Ella. He obviously believed that if Mark Ella was my preferred 5/8, there was no room for him.

I rather bluntly and impatiently ensured him to stop worrying, he would be in the team. And I dropped the remarkably gifted Australian vice-captain Michael Hawker, shifted Michael Lynagh out of position and played him at inside centre. His adjustment to a new role was extraordinary and he was a significant part of that historic Grand Slam success.

It was not without its moments. He was young. He'd absorbed a lot of pressure. I sensed after the Ireland Test that I should relieve him of goal-kicking duties. We were, of all things, shopping for Waterford crystal in Ireland. We were queued up and I told him, as we stood in the queue, that I was taking him off the goal-kicking duties for the Test against Wales.

Michael being Michael immediately assumed he was being dropped. I became impatient with his insecurity and told him that never under my watch would he be dropped. It was just that the great Roger Gould would assume goal-kicking duties.

Michael had a magnificent match, Roger Gould kicked to perfection and we set a record against Wales at Cardiff Arms Park. And more success was to follow, where this gifted and modest young Queenslander was a central component to our success.

We'd brilliantly won the Hong Kong Sevens, then the world championship of Sevens rugby in Sydney. We won a Test series in New Zealand in 1986—the only side, apart from the British Lions, ever to have achieved that. The '86 Wallabies won the deciding Test at Eden Park after a harrowing tour across the country by comprehensively defeating the All Blacks in the third Test. In drizzly conditions, Michael Lynagh's guts and skill were outstanding. And that '86 side was the last Australian side to beat New Zealand at Eden Park.

I feel privileged that Michael Lynagh and I still correspond regularly, to this day. We are, it's fair to say, closer now than we were then as coach and player. We rallied when we all took fright in 2012 when we learnt that Michael had suffered a stroke. But even then Michael Lynagh was the architect of his own triumph over adversity. He could have yielded to peer pressure when he felt that something had happened and pretended, macho like, that all was okay. Instead, he asked his mates to call for an ambulance immediately. It most probably saved his life. And what a life it's been to date.

I write to him regularly. I remind him that Australian rugby will never be able to repay the debt it owes to him. And yet beyond his extraordinary gifts is an extraordinary human being. I always told my players that it wasn't so very difficult to be a good player, but it was exceedingly difficult to be a good person. Michael Lynagh is such a person.

His great personal qualities derive, primarily, from the strength of his family ties and from the discipline and Christian teachings of his Alma Mater, St Joseph's College on Gregory Terrace in Brisbane.

In the manuscript of life, it is the little things that are indelible. I can't talk about Michael Lynagh without thinking about his Mum, Marie. She was a school teacher. All parents want to see their children walk across the international stage. So it was with Michael's parents, Ian and Marie.

I remember often visiting Marie and she'd be ironing for the family. But while she did, in the oven there'd be things like banana cakes and carrot cakes, which Marie would then sell to the local delicatessen. And all those monies went into a little kitty, which enabled her to, thankfully, be present for her son's greatest sporting triumphs.

This biography ploughs all that fertile ground again. It tells the story of an ordinary young boy from Queensland who, at an early age, did extraordinary things to become one of the greats of Australian sport.

Wherever the history of Australian rugby is written, the name of Michael Lynagh will always occupy a prominent place. But as I often say, long after the scoreboard is forgotten, the friendships remain. Our friendships with Michael are a consequence of him being, not a great rugby player or a splendid athlete, but rather of being a decent, modest, sharing and loving friend.

Books of this kind must be written. They offer a signpost for young people of tomorrow as to how talent is identified and success secured. There can be no more indelible proof of the challenge and excitement of the journey towards making something of your God-given gifts than is revealed in this story of Michael Lynagh.

Those of us who've played a small part in that story are immensely grateful that someone like this young man entered our lives and shared something with us in return.

We are forever in his debt.

Alan Jones AO
Broadcaster and Former Australian Rugby Union Coach

A NOTE FROM THE CO-AUTHOR

WHEN I WAS BUT a fourteen-year-old schoolboy in 1984, Michael Lynagh's existence was nothing more than a source of irritation for me. Scotland had won their own Grand Slam that year, and, delusional as it now may sound, there was a feeling among the Scots supporters that the touring Wallabies would not provide any sterner test than the Home Nations had. But by the time the Wallabies arrived at Murrayfield on December 8th 1984, the landscape had changed considerably. They'd soundly beaten everyone else.

As if tries being run in from every conceivable position by the likes of Ella and Campese wasn't misery enough to watch from the schoolboy enclosure, it was perhaps more frustrating to know that Lynagh, when presented with a kick from anywhere on the pitch, was almost certain to convert it. He kicked an Australian record that day. The respect I had for his ability was huge—if just a little grudging in a deeply patriotic sense.

From that day on, as he became increasingly synonymous with both excellent rugby and total humility, I could only admire Michael Lynagh's career, specifically the way in which he always put the game of rugby first and himself a distant second. He still does.

When I heard about his stroke in 2012, I was driving. I'd recently returned to visit family in Scotland and the car radio told the story: 'Wallaby great Michael Lynagh in a critical condition following a stroke.'

I had to pull over.

The fact that someone so young and healthy—so seemingly *invincible* in my eyes—had suffered a stroke really hit me hard. I felt physically sick. The other part that jolted me was acknowledging that Michael was only a few years older than me. That made me suddenly question my own mortality in a way I never had before.

A year or so later I made contact—'How about writing a book about your experiences? It could be a really inspiring message.'

'Ah, mate, I don't know. Would anyone care about what I have to say nowadays?'

Even after his traumatic life-changing experience, Michael Lynagh was as self-deprecating as he'd always been. He's also as loyal and as honest as anyone you could ever meet. It also took him almost two years to tell me that he's half-Scottish!

'Think about it,' I said.

He did. *Blindsided* is the result.

Mark Eglinton

For my family: my special wife Isabella and my beautiful sons Louis, Thomas and Nicolo. Also to my parents, Ian & Marie, and my sister Jane. Thank you all for always being there when I needed you and for being the reason I am still here.
Love Michael.

ONE

A VITAL DECISION

*Intensive Care Unit of the Royal Brisbane and
Women's Hospital, April 2012*

IT WAS PITCH BLACK and that was my choice. Via an uncomfortable process of elimination, I'd discovered that if I kept my eyes closed, somehow the pain in them lessened—the opposite to what I'd expected. The crushing pain in my head was much harder to dismiss, though. My head was screaming. Not aching—*screaming*. My cerebellum was swollen, pressing down to within fractions of millimetres of my brainstem. I could almost feel it straining within the confines of my skull. Any contact would be catastrophic.

I've been blindsided by a few big hits from back-row forwards over the years—the Mark Shaws and Eric Champs of this world have clobbered me a few times. No amount of tactical awareness or raw, self-preserving instinct could avert those. Sometimes you're just going to get hit. No warning, just a sudden and painful impact. Blindside hits are always the worst. You don't see them coming. But it's all part of what you sign up for when you play rugby at the highest level. This was real pain. And I hadn't seen it coming either.

As I lay in my hospital bed hooked up to all kinds of monitors—my bedclothes drenched with sweat, yet my bones frozen to their core—I was presented with the most important decision I would ever have to make. This was a choice far tougher than whether to keep the ball in play or kick for the corner; pass or make a cut inside a fast-closing centre: I had to decide whether I had the strength and desire to continue living. It was a profound moment.

It occurred to me right then that almost every facet of life, much like a game of rugby, boils down to decisions made at critical moments. The obvious difference being that a wrong call on the field might lose you the game, whereas in life's case, choices can have a much more far-reaching effect.

Given my awful predicament, the calmness with which I was able to evaluate the situation shocks me a little when I consider it now. First, I thought about my loving wife, Isabella. 'She'll be okay,' I admitted to myself. Let's face it—as much as we were in love and she meant the world to me, she was still pretty young with a long life ahead of her.

Then I turned my attention to my three boys: Louis, Thomas and Nicolo. I flinched inwardly for a moment as I considered the prospect of them growing up without me. Without a dad. But as hard as it was to accept, I had to acknowledge that they'd ultimately be fine too. Yes, in time, without me—Michael, Dad—everyone would be all right. Their lives would go on. That was reality.

It seemed so strange to be thinking in this cold, pragmatic way, and for someone as intrinsically positive as I am it was certainly a barometer of how exhausted I was. And of how much my brain hurt. It was as if I'd become detached from my addled mind and exhausted body and was a mere stranger looking at my situation from a purely practical perspective: 'This is how it will be.'

Maybe it was easier that way? After all, to remove emotion from the equation would certainly make my decision more straightforward, and that, at that precise moment, was perhaps what I needed. Selfishly, I just wanted no more pain and relief from my seemingly endless exhaustion. It might sound weak, but I was just too tired to keep going.

It also occurred to me that I'd had a really good life. I'd played top-level rugby successfully, worked in great jobs and, most importantly, had a wonderful family and a wide circle of true friends; I was very lucky. Part of me thought, 'This isn't where I want it to end, but if it has to, I can't really complain.' I'd reached that point.

Something was distracting me from this strange feeling of resignation, though. Initially it was irritating, but then it focused my mind and made me a little curious. In retrospect, it seems to me that because my vision was impaired, my sense of hearing had been greatly enhanced, as if to compensate.

Consequently, I had a heightened awareness of the continual, chaotic noise in the space around me, mostly made by the many machines I was attached to. Rest was impossible, given the loudness of the racket, and it began to really bug me— to the point where I vaguely remember asking if the machines could somehow be turned down. But the nursing staff told me that the alarms were necessary and that they weren't actually very loud anyway.

But as day merged with night and the unrelenting headache and the morphine drip forced me in and out of fitful sleep, I gradually became aware of some kind of order within the background cacophony. I had to focus hard to identify it, but when it came to me it seemed really obvious.

'That's Canned Heat,' I said to myself.

It was almost comical in its incongruity. I like the song; it's really catchy.

'Why this song and why here?'

In my head, the sounds of all the bells and whistles were combining, again and again, to mimic the short flute intro to the song 'Going up the Country'. Somehow their pitch and tone and the order in which each noise was produced by an alarm, sensor or monitor kept that two or three-bar musical motif looping round and round all day and night. I was pleased with myself that I'd managed to figure it out. Of course the song itself wasn't important. But the fact that it was *a song* was. It reminded me that the world I used to inhabit was still there, albeit a little out of reach for the time being.

But it *was* there.

More importantly, so was everything and everybody that mattered to me: my wife, my children, my parents, my friends; everything that I do and am … everything that I live for.

'I'm getting out of here; I want to see my kids again.'

Suddenly I had made my decision.

What on earth had I been thinking?

Me?

Giving up?

Not a chance.

One thing I had never been was a slacker—and I've never been one for self-pity. In my head I'd gone to that place of giving up and made a choice that it wasn't for me. Giving up wasn't me at all. I'd always faced situations head on, good or bad, and searched for the best way forward. If a situation was getting to me or wearing me down, I usually found a way to seize back control. I'd been that way since I was a young kid growing up in Queensland: on a surfboard, in business and with rugby ball in hand.

I decided to engage the proven mind-set that had guided my life and career: to dictate what happened next with my thoughts and attitude—'*This* is the way this is going to go.' The alternative didn't bear thinking about. Its cautionary voice in my head chastised me into action.

Seriously, mate, do you really want to die here, miles from home and not see your wife and children ever again?

Sound good?

Oh and by the way, you'll never play golf again, host a family barbecue or taste a glass of your favourite red wine. Are you fine with that too?

I cut the voice off before it went any further.

'Stop! No.'

The prospect of not experiencing those scenarios again, not to mention many others, was suddenly unthinkable. So there was no choice but to decide, there and then, that it absolutely wasn't going to happen. I was forty-eight years old, for goodness sake, and, until recently, as fit and healthy as any guy my age. Also, I had far too much still to do—much more to enjoy and achieve in my life. It was also gradually dawning on me how lucky I was to even have a choice as to what my next move was. After all, many people in my situation don't get that luxury; the option of life is just removed from the table for them.

So instead of thinking negatively, based on the pain, discomfort and frustration I felt, I turned it all around. 'All right, I'm in charge now.'

Because of the way I felt—the headache, the fatigue, the freezing cold, the confusion as to what the future held—I used what I didn't want, how I *didn't* want to feel, as my motivation. I wanted my life back.

TWO

TRANSCENDING NODDY

WRITING A BOOK CERTAINLY wasn't foremost in my mind in the latter part of 2012. First, an authorised biography of me, entitled *Noddy*—written by my friend and former Wallaby teammate, Andrew Slack—already existed, having been published in 1995. Incidentally, the nickname Noddy is one I've had since I was ten. A kid I was at school with fell asleep in class one day and I called him Noddy because he'd nodded off. He didn't like it and said, 'How would *you* like to be called Noddy?' And the nickname stuck.

As far as I was concerned, *Noddy* was a great book that had been received well, so what more could possibly be added? I stood back from the idea and thought, quite justifiably, 'Slacky did a great job.'

But then I thought about what was actually in the book: it only covered my life up to the year or so prior to the 1995 World Cup in South Africa, which was perhaps the tipping point of the biggest shift in the history of rugby union, with professionalism only months away. I'd never really considered that I was one of the few top-level players to have straddled the two eras of the game. Maybe, by doing so, I had a unique point of view to share?

Not just that; *Noddy* had covered those pre-professional years from a third-person point of view, albeit with considerable input from me.

I suppose that with the passage of time and all that it involved—marriage, kids, work and life generally—I had forgotten how long ago my playing career was. I certainly hadn't factored in that key element called perspective.

Measuring yourself during and after rugby—it's not easy. For years you strive to be a rugby player. Then you make it. You're like a performer every weekend. You're praised when you win and criticised when you falter. Then it's gone. You lose your identity. You feel like you're starting out again. It shouldn't be a surprise, because when you begin to play rugby, you know it's probably going to be over by the time you're thirty-five. You know that, but your mind will tell you lies anyway. Because there's always that fear of saying to yourself: 'This is it. My last game.'

Once you walk away from playing, you have to work out what you want to do with your life. It can be exciting—'What's coming next?' But part of me always knew that whatever I did post-rugby, it might not measure up to playing for Australia.

So after leaving hospital I began to think about the rugby days again. I transported myself back there to see how it felt. In my head I lost a few pounds, trimmed off the grey hairs and put myself back on the paddock in the green and gold—'I remember this place.'

Gradually I began to question whether what I'd felt back then accurately reflected how I feel now, and so, as the idea of writing this book was discussed in more depth with those closest to me, I started to believe that it might indeed be an interesting exercise to look back on certain aspects of my life from the point of view of a 48-year-old man—the guy you see with the glasses and the suit on Sky television, not the lithe, rugby-playing me of almost twenty years ago. Furthermore, I was a 48-year-old man who'd just survived a major stroke. A hell of a lot had changed. Aspects of my personality have been altered forever.

In those terms the idea of a new book seemed much more palatable. But I'd be lying if I said that I didn't still have some lingering reservations.

'How much do I really remember?'

'Will it be interesting even if I do?'

I also thought, 'Who would care about what I have to say nowadays?' The bottom line, too, is that I'm not someone who enjoys blowing my own trumpet. 'Look at me—I did all this great stuff all those years ago.' That's not my style. I'm also not a person who particularly likes delving into my emotions— far less putting them on show for the benefit of a worldwide reading audience. That's just not my personality.

Or at least I thought it wasn't.

But as I navigated the difficult few months after my stroke, my feelings began to change. I had to start measuring myself all over again, with a new set of standards based on my reduced vision. Inevitably I ran into all kinds of people who'd had similar or far worse experiences and outcomes than I'd had. I couldn't help but be profoundly moved by their stories. I met young people whose lives had been completely destroyed by stroke: everyday people who'd lost their job, home, a relationship—or maybe all three. Perhaps they'd become completely blind or were facing a permanent, life-altering physical disability.

These encounters focused my mind on two things. First, given the nature and severity of my own stroke, I acknowledged that I was incredibly lucky to be alive and in relatively good health. Though my vision was significantly impaired and there were adjustments to make as a result, I was still able to go to work, earn a living and be an active part of my family. Yes, it was tough at times on the emotional and physical fronts, but I'm still here and I'm increasingly grateful for that. As I compared myself to some of the people I met who'd also suffered strokes, I would be thinking, 'Jeez, I really dodged a bullet here.'

Secondly, I wanted to use my experiences and outreach to give something back to people who weren't in such good shape—people who needed something as basic as a reason to get out of bed each morning. These thoughts would develop, and are still developing as I write this. Life for me has always been an exercise in setting small goals. It's all very well having a grand dream, but I've always thought it's more important to plot how you're going to get there.

I started to look at the book idea from a different standpoint. The focus shifted away from me towards others. What about other people who'd had a stroke? What of the unfortunates who might have one someday down the line? Could my story benefit them in some small way? Perhaps a tiny aspect of how I approached recovery could be inspiring to them or their families, who bear the impact also. I've been around long enough to know that people who are in the public eye, even on the relatively small level that I am, have the ability to make a difference.

I wanted to make a difference.

That was a significant motivation behind this book.

Also, from a purely rugby perspective, there's an awful lot within those playing years that I've never actually *thought* about. Even in the burning heart of my career, I never dwelled on games or the incidents within them for very long, so I was interested to see how I'd view things today—through eyes that are a little wiser and more pragmatic, maybe. As I took a step back from the way I'd previously viewed my career I was surprised by what I saw.

Obviously, the game has changed hugely in the almost twenty years since I stopped playing in 1998. My position within the game has changed a lot too. Although my involvement with the sport has continued, albeit on the media side via my work for Sky Sports and other broadcasters, you can never recapture the emotions that you feel within the white lines of a playing field, no matter how many Super Twelve/Fourteen/Fifteen or Heineken Cup games you analyse from the comfort of the studio on a Saturday morning with Fitzy and the lads.

What I *can* do now is be both a bit more thoughtful and also outspoken about how events panned out while I was playing. It's not that I was deceiving myself or anyone else at the time; it was more a case of my preserving a poker-faced demeanour in my playing days, designed to deflect forces of negativity from both the outside world and, more crucially, from within *me*. There was also the Wallaby code of integrity and sportsmanship to promote, and I still hold that dear.

Although I probably never showed it in interviews or, for that matter, on the field, strong emotions *were* there, trust me.

It was just much easier to suppress them until some unspecified and distant day in the future than to deal with them at the time. I doubt I'm the first sportsman to process things that way. Maybe it's a bit old-fashioned, but it was the only way I knew. I always thought, 'You'll be fine if you just keep it all in, mate. Don't let anyone see that you feel.'

Now, that distant, unspecified day in the future has arrived. I've matured enough to have reconciled many aspects of my career and I'm in a position to speak about things a bit more openly than I ever was previously.

From a stylistic point of view, I should say that the idea of discussing every detail of my life and career in a chapter-and-verse 'I was born in Brisbane on October 25th 1963' way doesn't appeal to me. This book will not do that. While there will obviously be some crossover, *Noddy* has already covered a lot of that ground and done so very well. Instead, I want to be a little more selective and focus on a few aspects of my career, ones that best illustrate who I was, who I am now and how it all ties together.

Most of all, my life has been about committed decisions. They crop up almost every day and you've got to face them, armed with all the information you have at your disposal. That's the best you can possibly do in life. The rest is down to the intangibles that you just can't prepare for—and I've got experience of those.

THREE

THE ENDLESS ORDEAL

MANY PEOPLE ADVISED ME to read Andre Agassi's memoir *Open*, and when I did I was amazed, as most readers probably were, to learn that he as often as not hated the game of tennis. By any standards it was a pretty incredible admission. How could someone so successful and seemingly so driven have such a deep dislike for what he did best? The fact that he gave no indication of the way he felt when he was playing only made the admission more surprising. On most levels it just didn't make sense.

But when I thought more about it, I could understand, at least on a minuscule level, how he felt. I would never say, 'Actually folks, I always hated footie,' as, by and large, I loved the game and I still do. But I was always aware that it got in the way of a few things in life and I definitely made sacrifices over the years because of it. For example, in the early days, while a lot of my university friends might have been going camping or surfing at the weekends, I always had a game on a Saturday and would also have to train for it during the week prior. I don't now consider it a huge sacrifice, given what I got out of rugby in the long run; it's just a different choice that I made. It almost wasn't even a choice; it just happened.

More than anything, though, for a lot of the time it was the goal-kicking that was an absolute ordeal for me. The physical act was fine, but the fear of it not working always ate away at me mentally. In fact, I'll take that a stage further by saying that I've thought many times since retiring that if it wasn't for goal-kicking—and the psychological pressure that goes hand in hand with it—my career could have been extended. Not by much, but certainly by a couple more years.

I always knew that I felt the way I did, but I guess we all find coping mechanisms to deal with our fears or to block them out. I certainly never discussed my feelings with players or coaches, not even in the darkest moments. I always wanted to appear in control. 'Lynagh's so cool and measured,' commentators always said. That was news to me. Really, I was like a swan. I looked graceful, in control. Cruising on the surface. But underneath the water, in my head, there was always a hell of a lot going on.

My so-called quiet mind just isn't as quiet as most people's. My dad—a clinical psychologist—always said I was 'thoughty', particularly when I wasn't meant to be thinking at all. I thought about everything, and goal-kicking was just one of those things. I even remember sitting and crying to myself before games when I was younger, simply because I couldn't cope with my nerves.

With hindsight, the goal-kicking pressure was cumulative. It gnawed away in the back of my mind from my first under-12 games at school, all the way through to the end of my career. I didn't always notice or acknowledge the stress, of course, certainly not in my carefree younger days. But as my playing career moved into its final phase and the stakes got higher with the onset of professional rugby, I became increasingly aware of the mental hardship I was heaping on myself before, during and after games.

No wonder. The margin between success and failure, win and loss, was always such a small one. Consequently, I became increasingly conscious that points and percentages were the only two tangible measures of a goal-kicker's worth.

Anyone could look at a newspaper or a TV screen and say, 'Lynagh kicked well today', or equally, 'Lynagh had a shocker.' Those numbers did not lie. But what people couldn't possibly see was what I went through to kick either five from five or nought from seven. It took me a long time to even acknowledge that the statistics were a focus of agonising scrutiny from which there was simply no hiding place.

This responsibility and weight of expectation was apparent to me at Saracens, the professional club in north-west London that I joined in 1996, in particular. Nobody was putting it on me or expecting anything that they hadn't before. I was doing it to myself. I was always measuring myself. What had changed? What's the difference between, say, Saracens versus Leicester on a wet Saturday in February and any one of my 72 caps for Australia?

Well, first and foremost, by 1996 rugby had become a professional sport and goal-kicking was no longer just about points on the board. A number of my fellow players and friends were on win bonuses, which involved significant sums of money. So, in my mind, my role as the flyhalf and the goal-kicker became one on which much depended. I felt the weight immediately. I needed to respond to it. I wanted to make sure I did everything I could to win these matches for my team. I didn't get paid bonuses on a game-by-game basis myself—not unless we won a final or won the premiership. But it was still a huge responsibility knowing how much influence my kicks had not only on results, but also on livelihoods, the ability to pay mortgages and school fees. It was a new kind of pressure.

What was I going to do about it?

The key was preparation. During the last few years of my international career, I'd begun to scratch the surface of advanced preparation. Sometimes it worked; other times it didn't. But by experimenting, albeit on a relatively minor level, I'd learned that by identifying variables and making adjustments to account for them, goal-kicking became less of a lottery. It would never be an exact science, I knew that, but at least I could load the odds a little more in my favour.

My anxiety about kicking successfully at Saracens was the manifestation of years of mental anguish. The only way I could combat it was to prepare even better than I had ever done before. So I made it my business to get to the ground we were due to be playing at the day before the match, whenever it was feasible, so I could practise goal-kicking, line kicking, restarts—the whole gambit of what I do as the team kicker. I'd dabbled in this sort of preparation in the past, but never to this degree.

I'd practise right-sided restarts and left-sided restarts. Goal kicks into the wind, against the wind and across the wind. Line kicks up and down both touchlines and into all four corners. I'd watch how every ball behaved and take mental note—'That corner's a bit softer than this one.'

By practising, I became extremely familiar with the conditions that any particular environment might throw at me. So when it came to match day there was barely a scenario that I hadn't envisaged mentally and practised in reality many times. This level of preparation didn't take the fear away completely, but it at least tamed it and made me think, in each game-day situation, 'I've seen you before. I know what to do here.'

But still it was a challenge. Rugby venues, particularly club grounds, are all very different. On paper the dimensions of a rugby pitch are basically the same. But in reality, no two grounds are alike.

Different grass.

Different pitch dimensions.

Different wind directions.

Different visual sightlines.

Different lots of things: advertising hoardings, the colours of the letters on the advertising hoardings, the size and colour of the flags on the roof of the stands, and so on.

It might sound a little obsessive, but I had to know exactly what the differences were in advance, and, by extension, how they might affect my ability to kick an oval ball between the posts. That way I'd eliminate any variables for match day and, as a result, would be that little bit better prepared. All I wanted was to kick more goals.

Say we were playing Bristol on a Saturday. I'd ask our manager at some point during the week: 'Can you ring Bristol and tell them that I'll be down there at 3.00pm on Friday to practise goal-kicking?'

He'd go, 'No problem, I'll call them now.'

As far as was possible and practical, it became a part of my weekly routine—no matter where we happened to be playing. I'd drive myself down to Ashton Gate, say, in my car and at my expense, on the Friday afternoon, while the rest of the team would be coming down later in the bus. I did this off my own bat; nobody told me to do it and I never made a big fuss about it. I didn't get paid any extra, but I saw it as my responsibility and I did it—that's the game. That was *my* game.

My teammates saw what I was doing. They never said anything and, frankly, there was nothing to say. From my perspective, I didn't need them to comment. It wasn't about affirmation. It was about taking responsibility. Now I'm sure a few of them might have thought that worrying about their bonuses was something I didn't need to shoulder. But they didn't know that this approach was as much for my benefit as it was for theirs. I just needed them to know how much being prepared meant to me, and I'm sure, in their eyes, that was never in doubt. I was part of the team, trying to win games for the team. It was so important to me that I had the respect of the guys and that they never, ever, questioned my commitment.

Sadly, back in those fledgling professional days, there were more than a few players with a similar profile to me who turned up at clubs just to get paid and went home afterwards without putting in their best effort—'Thanks very much, that'll do nicely.'

I never wanted to be lumped into that category. I was always thinking the opposite: 'I'm not here for a free ride.' It's not a surprise then that nowadays every goal-kicker does what I did—it's actually considered part of the job. Back in 1996, it wasn't part of the job at all.

BACK IN THE AMATEUR era, when I played the majority of my rugby, it wasn't just goal-kicking practice that was taken a lot less seriously. Every aspect of the game was practised less. In the very early days, goal-kicking wasn't something I worked on much and that itself was a problem I should have identified at the time. I was all about feel and—with hindsight—I probably always underestimated just how much natural ability I had. I relied on it and anything else—practice, mental preparation etc—was just a bonus. I wasn't giving it more thought than most kickers, but with hindsight, I probably should have practised more.

People always said I was too hard on myself. I don't agree with that. Maybe I just expected—demanded—more of myself than most, and, looking back, it's possible that I was aiming for things that simply weren't realistic in terms of kicking goals. But I didn't look at it like that at the time. As far as I was concerned, I was just doing my very best for every team I represented.

As amateur rugby players, we worked all day in our real jobs or perhaps studied at university, as I did. The emphasis was completely different. Rugby was secondary then. After uni I worked in property and that didn't leave a lot of time once I'd done my nine to five and then been to training in the evening. The last thing I wanted to do was practise kicking after I'd worked all day and then driven across Brisbane to train from six until eight-thirty at Ballymore. I could only do so much in a day.

That said, on the occasions when goal-kicking wasn't working for me, and there were certainly a few, I did try to fix the problem. But not in what you'd call a scientific way. I'd just stand in front of the posts and kick a few to see if I could get the feeling of knocking them over back. Even in games on the weekend, it was a case of just seeing how it went rather than knowing what to do and what to adjust. Thinking about it makes the task of kicking successfully even more stressful, because 'feel' isn't tangible. There's no reason why you have it one moment and not the next.

So for the first three-quarters of my career, at Queensland and even for Australia, back in the amateur 1980s and early 1990s, a lot depended on unquantifiable things like 'feel' and momentum. Because I didn't practise enough, most of my stress was brought on simply by my not knowing which me would turn up—the ace goal-kicker or the hopeless one. 'I wonder how it's going to go *this* weekend,' was my persistent worry.

I liken the feeling to stepping onto the first tee when you haven't practised your golf for a while. You think things like, 'God, I hope I don't hook this out of bounds', all the while knowing that hoping probably isn't going to be enough. I've been in a few situations on golf courses where I could barely draw the club back on the first tee. I remember standing on the first tee at St Andrews, playing in the Alfred Dunhill Challenge with Adam Scott. It's a huge fairway; it's almost impossible to miss it. But if you haven't been practising or have the yips, it's easy to do. Just ask Ian Baker-Finch.

When I finally poked it out there I said, 'Thank God that's over.' Adam Scott said, 'You've played in front of 80,000 people. What's the problem?' I said, 'Mate, at least at Twickenham, I know what I'm doing. Out here, it can go anywhere.' That's a bit what it felt like being an amateur rugby player. By and large, my kicks could go anywhere.

Everything usually hinged on my first kick. If I got a hard kick out on the touchline and missed it, all of a sudden I might find myself none from two, even if the second kick was from an easier position. From there I'd be behind the proverbial eight ball. Getting tense. Trying too hard. Probably making mistakes in an effort to get the scoreboard ticking over. Equally, if I slotted that first one from the touchline, I usually thought, 'Okay, I'm in business. Here we go ...'

When everything felt great, I could carry the positivity with me from there through the game. Kicks immediately seemed easier. Confidence definitely fuelled success. But, conversely, lack of it could consume me very quickly. It didn't take much for the doubts to start creeping in.

I'm sure I wasn't alone in this situation. Back in the 1980s and '90s it's unlikely that any one kicker was doing a huge amount of practice. I know I wasn't. There just wasn't room in the amateur player's life to dedicate to it and my perception was that I wasn't doing any more than most. When I was at a low ebb, I used to occasionally wonder if anyone else was putting extra work in to gain an advantage. I used to lie in bed at night and think, 'I wonder if Foxy's putting extra hours in?' I never asked him, though. I don't think anyone really thought about it, far less discussed it.

GRANT FOX, FORMER ALL BLACK FLYHALF: I wasn't as diligent in the early days as Michael was. The danger of trying to seek perfection is that you tend to overthink things. You get paralysis by analysis. When you think about it, goal-kicking isn't that hard. I tried to view it like that for the first few years.

The result of this lack of focused practice and the associated confidence rollercoaster was that, unless all my kicks were right in front of the posts, a 70 per cent success rate was considered a good day for me in the early years. I'd be happy with that. In contrast, in my professional days at Saracens, if I'd kicked at 60 per cent, I'd soon have been sitting on my backside in the stand on weekends, watching someone else take shots at goal. My strike rate at Saracens was much closer to 80 per cent because I'd done all the homework I possibly could. I was an older man but I was a much better goal-kicker. I approached the discipline completely differently. But I'd started thinking about how I might do that long before I became a professional.

AS THERE OFTEN IS, there was a specific turning point in my attitude to goal-kicking and how best to prepare for it—a single watershed event that triggered an 'I need to rethink *everything* that I'm doing' epiphany.

It came a full seven years into my international career: at Eden Park, Auckland, on August 24th 1991. Australia had won the first game of the Bledisloe Cup series in Sydney 21–9. It wasn't really as close as that. We'd played very well. Another win or, crucially, even a draw would be enough for us to regain the trophy.

GRANT FOX: The game in Sydney is the only time in my entire career where I was standing there thinking, 'We can't win this game.' I almost felt helpless. Even later, in the 1991 World Cup semi-final in Dublin, I always felt that we were capable of winning. But in Sydney I felt, 'Christ we're just hanging on here.' We got beaten 21–9 and we were lucky to get that bloody close.

I'd kicked five from five in Sydney. I had every right to feel pretty confident about how I was striking the ball. The positive momentum was there. I was right in the zone. While I knew full well that it wasn't a permanent state, at least I was there. Not just that: there was a growing sense among the team that we'd crossed a line as far as the All Blacks were concerned. We felt that by beating them in Wellington a year previously we had removed an invisible ceiling. Of course they were still strong, by any standards. A bad All Black team is a contradiction in terms. But the 1991 All Blacks were an ageing team with several of their top players in the twilight of their careers. Guys like Kieran Crowley, Steve McDowall and Terry Wright were all great players, but closer to the end of their careers than to the beginning.

Matching them physically was one thing, and we certainly did that. It was almost as if our forwards decided, after the disappointments of the 1987 World Cup, 'Teams might be better than us technically, but we'll dig deep and take it to them. Hard.' Tommy Lawton, Simon Poidevin—they were big, physical presences who thought nothing of laying their bodies on the line on every possession. These forwards seemed to elevate their commitment to a new level and it was winning us games that we hadn't been winning before.

On the psychological side you also have to know that you can beat the All Blacks. It was always tough playing New Zealand. But if you competed with them rather than just accepting that they were the world's best, they became frustrated and tensed up. But first their opponents had to get over the psychological hurdle of the haka and the black jumpers, which they used as intimidation factors. A lot of teams would be ten points behind the All Blacks before the game even started, especially after letting the haka get under their skin.

In 1985, when I first faced it, I was a little intimidated by the haka too. But then I realised what it was and after that I don't have any real memories of it. I told myself, 'You know what it is: a dance, admittedly a war dance. You know they're going to do it and there's not much you can do about it.' You can either get worked up about it or you can let it happen.

I remember sitting on the bus with Nick Farr-Jones on the way back to the team's hotel after that first Bledisloe Cup match in Auckland in 1985. We'd lost the match 10–9. I looked at him and said, 'Mate, we really should have won that game, you know.' Nick agreed. Beforehand I'd been all worked up and nervous, thinking, 'But it's the All Blacks ...'

I realised only afterwards that they were just like anyone else. There was no need to get overcome by their aura. They used that aura and their traditions very well. I don't know if they're trained in it, but they do use it and it works if you let it. Nick and I agreed right then that we'd never bow to the fear factor again. We jointly thought, 'It's just a game of rugby; let's go out there and take them on from now on.'

To beat the All Blacks, you have to feel that there's no longer that aura to contend with, and all the team felt that we'd finally reached that place even prior to the first 1991 Bledisloe match in Sydney. I certainly thought, 'We might just have your number now, boys.'

But regardless of the psychological battles you win, you've still got to go out there and do it, on the pitch, and often in their back yard. That's never easy. It's all very well saying, 'We'd like to win this.' But you've got to think more about the small goals along the way. What area of the game did we need to focus on to achieve that ultimate goal of winning? Equally, which aspects of the game did we need to steer away from? It all had to be considered. And statistics said that we hadn't beaten the All Blacks at Eden Park since 1986 when a 22–9 victory in Auckland had given us a rare series win in New Zealand.

UNLIKE 1986, WHEN PLAYING conditions had been merely damp, Auckland was a wet, windy and pretty miserable place for rugby in August 1991.

It was a tense, disjointed match, attritional and non-expansive, with lots of dropped passes. There was frustration on both sides. Some pretty pedantic refereeing didn't help, if memory serves me well. There was so much on the line. Not only was the Bledisloe Cup at stake, but the winners would also carry considerable momentum (and likely favouritism) into the World Cup, to be held in the UK a couple of months later. That was the theory, anyway.

Unlike in Sydney, we were using what would be the World Cup ball. It was an early attempt at a synthetic ball and from the start it seemed as if each one behaved completely differently from any other. One would fly one way and the next would do more or less the opposite. No matter where on its surface you kicked it, the ball seemed strange. It was a goal-kicker's nightmare.

Consequently, the stats don't make great reading. Grant Fox missed a few kicks that day—that's unusual. Foxy was as close to a machine as you could get and knew Eden Park like his own front room. I was off target with a few too. But with less than a minute remaining—fifty-seven seconds, to be precise—we got a penalty, ten metres in from the left touchline. We were 6–3 down. This one would negate the missed ones. It would tie the game at 6–6 and give Australia the Bledisloe Cup. Most of the Wallaby team had never even touched the cup before.

GRANT FOX: We both had issues that day. It was wet, swirling winds—crap conditions, really. These were the early days of synthetic balls and they weren't the best balls to use. In those days, the home team got the last look at the ball, and if memory serves me correctly we over-inflated the ball that day—probably by a pound or a pound and a half. With the benefit of hindsight, the bloody thing had no hope of flying properly. We just had this thing that floated terribly—no forgiveness in it whatsoever.

Conventional wisdom suggests that the left side of the field is the favourable angle for right-footed, round-the-corner kickers. That was true for me. There was no technical reason to support that, though. It was more about comfort. The left side was just a more comfortable position from a visual perspective in that it looked natural for a round-the-corner kicker. No matter where I was on the field, though, I always tried to set the ball up exactly the same way before each kick, in spite of the fact that back in the days before kicking tees there were a lot more variables.

For example, contrary to how it probably looks on TV, pitches don't all have the same depth of grass cover. Where Twickenham might have had four or five inches of lush, green grass back then, somewhere like Ballymore in Brisbane—where they often had to drain the pitch with a pump because of the nearby creek and low water-table—might be bare in places, clumpy in others. That makes a big difference to not only how you create a platform upon which to place the ball, but also how your foot needs to connect with the ball. On a deeper surface, you need to make sure you get underneath the ball, whereas on a bare surface you can just kick it off the top.

Then there was the amount and consistency of the sand that was brought out to you by the ball boy to consider. If there wasn't enough, it was hard to build a sufficiently tall mound. If the sand was too dry and powdery, the kicking platform would simply fall apart and spread all over the grass. You never really knew what you were going to get and there were no rules to stipulate such things. So kicking was much less of an exact science than it is nowadays, when a plastic tee that's been tailored specifically for you means that, no matter where you are on any field, you're always kicking from exactly the same height. There's a lot less left to chance today.

Regardless of all the variables, I always tried to draw an imaginary line through the seam of the ball, and then tried to kick the ball right down that line towards the target. I suppose it's similar to how a golfer might imagine his swing path through the golf ball and towards the green or the hole. I'd visualise the path of my foot through the ball and extend that through its trajectory towards the posts. In theory, it's simple. In practice, it's less so.

Incidentally, that visualising approach went back a long way to conversations I'd had with my dad. He'd taught me the principles of mental rehearsal way back when I was a teenager. 'Think what you want to happen. Actually *see* it in your mind's eye.' That's what he'd tell me, and this was when sports psychology was in its infancy. 'Then when you've seen it, go and *do* it.'

IAN LYNAGH, MICHAEL'S FATHER, PSYCHOLOGIST: I didn't do a lot of formal stuff with Michael, but the early '80s was the early stages of sports psychology becoming a regular thing within high-profile sports. In 1983, I'd been made a consultant to the Australian Institute of Sport, and I also ran a private practice in Brisbane. This was when Michael was just starting his rugby career so the two coincided very well. Goal-kicking lent itself to quite a lot of mental control and mind-management strategies. I also helped with how to prepare mentally for a game. Michael quickly developed a whole routine of preparation and mental rehearsal for games and I know that he continued to run them his whole career. But this was very early days, particularly in the sport of rugby.

I always took Dad's advice very seriously. It worked for me. Even as a teenager I'd lie with my eyes closed in a warm bath at exactly 11am every match day, rehearsing in my mind what I was going to physically do later that day. It formed part of my ritual and it became an invaluable means of relaxing and allowing my mind to focus without interruption. Unbelievably, sports psychology was still an emerging concept in the early '80s.

Once I'd completed the visualisation process on the field, as my dad had instilled into me, I'd take four steps back and three to the left. Then came the calming words I said to myself over and over, hundreds of times.

Slow ... rhythm ... through.

Those words were important cues. First, they were my signal to clear my mind of peripheral thoughts. Secondly, they reminded me to switch over to the mode I needed to be in to kick effectively. I'd realised that most of the kicks that

I'd missed in games had failed because I'd tried to execute too quickly. When you think about it, kicking requires fine motor skills, but the combination of pressure and intense physical contact and exertion prior to the kick inevitably elevates your heart-rate and makes you speed up—it's basic physiology. So when starting my pre-kick routine, it was always important to remind myself to slow everything right down, almost to the point of exaggeration as if I was operating in slow motion.

Having gone through this tried and tested routine in Auckland, I stood motionless with that big grandstand behind me along the touchline, ready to kick the crucial three points. I'd seen it, now it was time to execute the vision.

I looked around Eden Park, felt the electric atmosphere. And the rain. There was a breeze too. The flags on top of the stand told me that. But because of the structure behind me, masking it at ground level, I couldn't physically feel it.

My right foot struck the seam of the ball exactly where I wanted it to. I was always a straight kicker—not a hooker or a slider of the ball like some other guys—and this one, despite the inconstancy of the ball, felt beautiful.

The ball took off, heading straight for the middle of the posts.

'Yeah,' I said to myself as the ball continued on its path, 'that looks good.'

You could hear a pin drop—35,000 people were holding their breath. I was one of them.

I was almost ready to turn away, as from a successful kick. Almost, but not quite.

Something didn't look right.

The plan was unravelling.

As the ball got closer to the goalposts and started to lose power—suddenly exposed to the elements as it passed from the shelter of the grandstand—a fresh gust of wind caught it at the last moment and pushed it just past the right upright.

I heard the dull thud as the ball hit the wet turf before the roar went up.

I had missed.

I was distraught—'How could that happen?'

We lost the game. The Bledisloe Cup would stay in New Zealand. No matter how often teammates told me, 'Mate, it's not your fault', or, 'Nah, we had plenty of other opportunities to win the game, mate', I didn't want to hear any of it.

BOB DWYER, FORMER AUSTRALIAN COACH: Foxy and Michael were great goal-kickers over a long period. When Foxy kicked the winning kick, he slipped and ended up flat on his back. That's how difficult it was. My view was: kickers don't lose you games. They can often win you them. To put it all on one guy is just too tough an assignment. We collectively were never of the opinion that he lost us that game. It's up to everyone to win the game and it's up to everyone to prevent the team from losing. But Michael had different standards that he imposed on himself.

I was so disappointed with myself. I hated excuses. I'd had a kick to tie the game and had missed it. It was as simple as that. Of little consolation was the fact that I had at least made good contact with the ball under extreme pressure. That part I had executed pretty well. But I knew there was wind and I hadn't factored it in. Poor planning. Rookie mistake.

GRANT FOX: I didn't really process the vagaries of a stadium as diligently as Michael did. And sometimes the odd stadium was just too hard to read. Then there's also that theory of 'A well-struck golf ball isn't affected by the wind', so sometimes you've got to trust that. Having said all that, I knew Eden Park like the back of my hand. I knew that there was a certain wind that might feel one way but it actually did something different. It was only through years of playing at Eden Park that I knew that. Michael would have probably had that relationship with places like Ballymore, or anywhere else he played a lot of games.

I felt like I needed to go back to the drawing board.

From that day on, I made a conscious decision to work far harder to improve the mechanics of my execution. But that was just half the commitment I made to myself. The other was to identify and, if possible, eliminate factors that might cause me to miss a kick, regardless of potential intangibles like the inconstancy of the ball. Wind, weather and all the various quirks a stadium might present—all needed to be accounted for. No two stadiums were the same, after all. Particularly in those days of low ends or sometimes even open ends. The wind would behave differently every time. You learn that from years of experience.

I kept thinking about the concept of preparation and decided that my commitment to prepare better wasn't something that should be exclusive to my rugby. It needed to apply to every part of my life: relationships and business as well as sport. I'd create small, attainable goals in life. Little milestones. I'd always look for a way to measure my progress.

When I reflect now, I realise that I definitely needed to freshen things up back then anyway. That's a natural response to a pivotal moment like missing a vital kick, I think: to change the routine. Alter something. I'd been doing the same thing for so long. It had been working. But suddenly it felt like it wasn't.

So though I retained the *slow ... rhythm ... through* aspect of my preparation, as that need to slow down would always apply, I found a slightly different way of getting to the same point in my pre-kick routine. It's like a tennis player who, instead of bouncing the ball four times before each serve, decides to bounce it only twice. It doesn't matter why—it's the change that counts. It has something like a placebo effect. You think you're getting a drug, but really you're not, yet you tell yourself—'That works. I feel better already!'

In the same way, a golfer might do something slightly different when addressing a putt, but would ultimately still strike the putt exactly the same way. Again, the details of the change don't really matter—it's the alteration in the routine that does. All of a sudden the putts start dropping again—'I've found the secret!'

So instead of taking the four steps back and three across, I made a mental note of where I would end up if I did that. Then I tried to find a new way of getting there, like walking backwards in an arc to that identical finishing point. It was such a simple thing. It initially felt alien, like writing with your weak hand. But it made a big difference in the place that mattered: my mind. It *felt* like I was doing something new, and goal-kicking, as much as it's a technical act, is also a lot about feel.

I'd have plenty of opportunity to put my new theories to the test.

FOUR

A RUGBY BAPTISM

PEOPLE HAVE COMMENTED THAT my eldest son, Louis, is a very nice, kind child. As his father, that's really nice to hear. Even though he's only fourteen, he has always had the ability to speak to adults in a polite way. To be fair, I've always been reasonably tough on him, but in a good way, I think. If he does something wrong, he knows it. But, by the same token, if he does something right he knows it as well. I think there's a balance to be found there. I don't start shouting and cheering just because he runs onto a rugby field. He needs to do something more than that before I start applauding.

You see far too much undeserved praise being heaped on kids these days—'Oh, my son's the *best*. You won't believe what he did today: he opened a can of fruit, all on his own. And I didn't have to help him. He's just such a wonderful, coordinated kid.'

I scratch my head and think, 'Come on?!'

That's just an example, of course, but, without wishing to generalise too much, most kids do the same things, albeit at slightly different ages. Don't give them praise for something that every kid can do, sooner or later. It's not fair on them in the long run. When they get out there into the real world, they'll find that they're not as great as they've been told all their lives. I'm of the opinion that kids should be left to be kids. By all means give them some guidance and help them along the way. But kids, by and large, will figure things out on their own.

I think my approach to parenting was inspired by my own dad, Ian. I've probably added a few tweaks of my own too. Dad was always extremely supportive of me when I was a child. He and my mother, Marie, were both invested in everything I did. It was definitely a loving relationship. But they didn't spoil me. Dad, particularly, was always very fair with praise when it was deserved. It wasn't given cheaply and I really respect that. You had to have done something well to get it, but in some ways that made life easier. You knew where you stood with Dad. If he praised you for something, you knew it was good. But on the other hand, he was always there to give me an encouraging talk or to help me with whatever it was that I was doing. He was certainly aware that, because I wasn't particularly confident as a child, part of his parental role was to help bolster my self-esteem. Both he and Mum were wonderful from that perspective.

Whatever I wanted to do, Dad would happily introduce me to it. When we lived on the Gold Coast, surfing was something I just loved. It all started when Mum and Dad bought me a surfboard for Christmas one year. They still joke about why they bought it for me in the first place.

Every Saturday and Sunday we used to go down to the beach. Mum and Dad would sit and relax and I'd swim out way beyond the breakers to try to catch a wave and bodysurf. A lot of times I'd get stuck out there and the lifeguards would come and rescue me. I was probably only six or seven at the time. The accepted signal for wanting to be rescued was to raise your hand, and I knew that. But sometimes I'd just raise my hand because I was waving to my parents on the beach. And then the lifeguards would come out. They probably thought, 'Not *you* again ...'

To me it was all good fun. My parents, on the other hand, thought: 'If he's going to keep going out beyond the breakers, we'd better get him a surfboard to hold on to.' So they bought me this terrible old thing. I remember it very clearly. It was orange underneath and green on top, with just a single fin. That was it for me, though. The board itself didn't really matter; I was hooked on surfing from that moment on.

At five-thirty or six every Saturday morning Dad would take me down to Burleigh Heads. Sometimes I'd say, 'Can we go down to Greenmount, or Snapper Rocks, or Kirra, Dad, where the really good waves are?' And he'd say, 'Yep', and off we'd go.

People always ask me, 'Did your Dad surf? Did he play rugby? Did he play cricket? Was he sporty?' I say 'No', and Dad hates it, because he did play rugby, he did play cricket and he did surf. He hates it even more when I say to him, 'Yeah, you were just a guy that played a bit of everything.' That's about the level that most people reach. There's nothing whatsoever wrong with that either.

But he was a better teacher than most. He understood the basics of most sports; he just couldn't do them very well! He had a lot of patience with me, though. When I wanted to go to the cricket nets to practise, *every single day*, he was pretty good at doing that and he did exactly the same for my sister, Jane, with whatever she was interested in at the time.

I should probably say that Jane and I are completely different types of people. We are poles apart. And that was sometimes a problem when we were growing up. I was always shy and reasonably introverted, without being anti-social. I had friends and got on with people, but I was quiet. Jane was loud and extroverted. She liked being the centre of attention, whereas I didn't like being in the spotlight. Nothing much has changed. If someone said, 'So you're Michael's sister?' Jane would say, 'No, he's *my* brother!' It was the same thing, of course, but with different emphasis.

She and I just pulled in different directions. Whereas I liked rock bands like the Rolling Stones and punk rock generally, she liked Abba. I hated Abba, although I've come to realise that Abba did what they did very well. But back then, they were like the antichrist. I used to think, 'If you like the stuff I like, you can't also like Abba.' We had different tastes in everything and that meant that we fought quite a lot.

As adults we obviously learned to get along a bit better. She's still outgoing and vivacious. Her industry is advertising and she's very good at it. It suits her personality perfectly. Advertising *isn't* my area—particularly when it relates to me. I'd always rather be in the background.

YOU'D PROBABLY BE SURPRISED to learn that rugby was not my main sport as I was growing up. My childhood was spent on the Gold Coast and we moved up to Brisbane in 1974, where my dad had a new job. Until that point I'd been playing soccer and a bit of rugby league at school. In those days, school rugby league was played by weight. So the teachers would say, 'Lynagh, you're stocky and pretty strong so you can play for the year above.' I was ten, playing with eleven- and twelve-year-olds. For me league was a pastime, nothing more.

Cricket was my main sport, my real love. I loved league and soccer but they were really just things that I did in the winter while waiting for the cricket season to come around again. But when we arrived in Brisbane in 1974, I discovered this game called rugby union at the school I went to: St Joseph's College.

Even when I was playing in the A team, running around a bit, I didn't really know the rules. I remember one day in particular. We were playing out at Nudgee College, our main rivals. Dad was there, as he was every Saturday for every sport I ever played. My parents *supported*—that's what they were great at. And they did it above and beyond the call of duty. They willingly took me to all my sports commitments every weekend. I saw that and do the same for my kids now.

'I want to play golf.'

'Okay, let's get you golf lessons.'

'I'd like to play tennis.'

'We'll take you to the tennis courts.'

It's in my nature to want to make sports, and opportunities generally, available to my kids. My parents did it for me and it encouraged me. I, in turn, do it for mine.

After this particular game at Nudgee, however, Dad was pretty quiet in the car on the way home. I didn't know what the problem was.

He said, 'If you're going to play this game, you've got to participate.'

I think he was frustrated because I was running around aimlessly, in his opinion.

'Either you get involved and learn the rules, or you go and do something else.'

I said, 'I want to play. I just don't understand the game very well.'

So I learned the rules, took the game more seriously and gradually rugby union became very important.

At my school, when you went from year seven into year eight (that is, primary school into high school), the class size doubled. New kids came in from the outside. We had rugby trial matches with all the new kids and I remember that I played in a reasonably weak trial team. I was playing flyhalf and spent most of the game in cover defence because we were getting beaten.

After the game, the coach, Brother Edwards, said, 'You're playing number eight from now on.' He was a good bloke, but he had obviously read somewhere that if you make a lot of cover tackles, you'd make a good number eight. I said, 'Well, I don't like playing number eight. I don't like getting involved in the scrums either.' But I got put in the under-13 B team anyway, playing number eight.

The next year, the under-14 coach said, 'You're not a number eight, you're playing flyhalf.' The following year I got into the First XV as a flyhalf. *That's* when it all happened. That's when it went from being recreational. Not just that, but I went straight into a team that had won the GPS Premiership two years running. We had a lot to live up to. Fortunately, I was coached by a very good schoolboys coach called Lester Hampson, and it was he who taught me a lot about the game generally and some of the skills particular to playing at number ten. His coaching was vital to me at that stage of my development.

While I mention this, it reminds me of a question I get asked a lot—'Who's your least favourite opposite number to play against?' You might assume that I'd nominate guys like Grant Fox, Rob Andrew and Hugo Porta. Actually, my least favourite was a guy called Rod Wilton. You won't have heard of him.

I came up against him while playing for St Joseph's at cricket and rugby at the under-13 level. He attended Nudgee. He was a batsman; I was a batsman. He was a flyhalf; I was a flyhalf. We both ended up in our respective First XVs and First XIs. He was a stocky country boy from Biloela in central Queensland and a smoker from the age of about fourteen, as I recall. I hated playing rugby against him because he was physically tough and very good. He remains my least favourite opponent.

Even though I was doing well at rugby, cricket was still my sporting passion. I played First XI at the age of thirteen and if you'd asked me, or my parents, which sport I was more likely to play for my country, the answer would definitely have been cricket. My cricket was miles ahead of my rugby.

Then circumstances intervened.

What decided my life's direction was that in 1981, my last year at school, an Australian Schools rugby team was selected to tour the UK in November and December. It would have been my first cricket season outside school. I went on tour instead. Life changed in an instant.

BOB DWYER: I used to live in a Sydney beach suburb called Coogee. My house was maybe a kilometre from the rugby ground. I was driving past one Saturday morning and I saw some teams playing. A friend of mine was coaching one of them ... the Australian Schoolboys. So I pulled over, watched the end of the game and when it was over I said to my friend, 'Who's the number ten?' He said, 'He's the star.' I said, 'Well, I've worked that out. What's his name?' And it was Michael. He stood out, even in a practice game when he was playing against nobodies. He had skill, balance, coordination and he was a very good kicker.

When I came back to Australia in January, I was selected for the Queensland senior rugby team and that was it. I never played cricket again until 1996, when I was invited to play in a few charity matches in the UK. I loved it, playing with people I'd grown up watching, like Derek Underwood, Barry Richards, Graeme Pollock and more recent Test players like Mark Butcher, Ashley Giles and Gladstone Small. It was surreal to have players like that down the other end. I thought to myself, 'I eventually made it as a cricketer—thirty years late!'

Before I knew it, my rugby career had started. Life was rolling forwards. I played my fourth game out of school for Queensland against a New Zealand select XV for the centenary of the Queensland Rugby Union in 1982. It was just my second game for Queensland and it was essentially against the All Blacks in everything but name. I was just a kid. I'd never played anybody. Man, we got run over in our own centenary game at home. It wasn't pretty.

There was a fellow from Wellington called Tu Wyllie playing at ten for the New Zealanders. He was a Maori, five foot ten and about fifteen or sixteen stone. He loved the Maori sidestep: straight over the top—'That'll teach you, you young little superstar.' He had huge thighs and charged over the top of me, all day long. That was the kind of flyhalf I didn't like.

On the other hand you have someone like Grant Fox. Foxy was a great player and was dangerous because he could run the game from a tactical perspective. But physical confrontation? Never.

I vividly remember a Bledisloe Cup match in Wellington in 1990. Because Grant wasn't commonly used as a runner, we always used to drift off him in anticipation of the ball going wider to the dangerous guys outside him. On this occasion, Grant got the ball and I drifted towards his inside centre as usual. But he saw me, held on to the ball and went for the gap inside me. I don't think Grant had ever scored a try in a Bledisloe Cup game and I remember thinking, 'Oh no, I hope he's not about to score because he's just gone inside me.' I didn't want to go down in history for that. I just managed to turn around, grab him by the shirt and drag him to the ground where a ruck formed on top of us.

As we were getting up off the ground as the play moved on, I accidentally stood on his hand. I said, 'Sorry mate, I didn't mean that.' Foxy said, 'No, don't worry, it's fine.' Here we were, two number tens apologising to each other as a Bledisloe Cup match raged around us. It was civilised. Our forwards would have been horrified to hear it. 'Let's not tell anyone about this,' we both agreed.

He and I were alike in that way: we didn't really relish physical confrontation. Grant was a terrific player, but guys like Rod Wilton and Tu Wyllie were completely different: they would run at you, make breaks against you and be very physical in doing so.

My quick baptism into Queensland rugby, straight from school, shows how a decision, even a small one, can make a huge difference to the direction of your life. I never really set out to play rugby for Australia, but in 1983 I did so against an Italian A side in L'Aquila. It was at night and it wasn't a particularly nice place to play. It was always a very difficult stadium to play at, as I'd find out in later years. Italian rugby wasn't the standard it is nowadays, but they weren't too bad. They had some good players who'd been around a little bit but we beat them pretty easily both in L'Aquila and later in Padova, where the Test was played, though I wasn't in the Test team.

My first real cap came against Fiji in Suva, in June of 1984. I played centre outside Mark Ella and it was in absolutely awful conditions. I hardly touched the ball. What was more interesting than that first cap in Suva was that I was dropped to the bench straight afterwards for the year's first Test against New Zealand at the Sydney Cricket Ground, which we won 16–9. David Campese and Mark Ella did the kicking and Michael Hawker took my place. The same team played at Ballymore two weeks later and the All Blacks won 19–15, setting up a decider at the Sydney Cricket Ground two weeks later.

In between, I played for Queensland against the tourists and we were run over 39–12, also at Ballymore. There was a pretty depressing mood in the dressing room afterwards, and just as I was leaving, the Wallaby coach, Alan Jones, came in and said he wanted to talk to me. He told me that he was thinking that the third All Black Test was one that required a really good goal-kicker.

Jones said, 'Would you play?'

I said, 'But where would you play me?'

He said, 'Don't worry about that, I'll take care of that part. But if you must know, I was thinking of playing you at fullback.' He thought that Mark Ella was playing well, and Michael Hawker was playing well at centre, but he thought I could replace Roger Gould, who was also playing well at the time, at fullback.

I told Alan that I thought I'd let the team down. I'd hardly ever played fullback and I was only nineteen, in my third year out of school. I think he was pretty taken aback, to be honest. I'm not sure he was used to people saying no to him. People always say, 'I'd play anywhere for my country', and that's true to some extent. But when you get faced with a situation where somebody you're supposed to replace is playing well, then I think it's fine to say what you feel. Roger was a far better fullback than me. That was a fact. He was proven; I wasn't. Thinking back recently it occurred to me, 'How many guys play in their first Test match in a big game and then never play again?'

In the end, they didn't pick me and it was absolutely the right decision. Campo and Mark Ella kicked most of their goals that day. Alan and I never discussed the matter again.

Even when I'd debuted for Australia, I never really thought I was that good. It just kind of happened and I went with it. But not to the exclusion of other things I enjoyed. Rugby has always been in perspective for me because I knew it was just one part of my life. No win meant so much to me that I got caught up in my own ego. That never happened, even after winning a World Cup.

Equally, no defeat plunged me so far into despair that I couldn't function day to day. Losses hurt, of course they did. But in the same way that a win was always made up of a series of moments that contributed towards an outcome, I gradually came to realise—via some tough lessons—that defeats are made up of similar components too. It was never just about one kick, just as life isn't all about one day.

And there was always next weekend. You live for next weekend. And, on a wider scale, when rugby was over, I knew that it was just one phase of my life. There was going to be a great life afterwards for me. I always knew that at the end the highs and lows would probably balance out. I think that attitude helped make my rugby career a lot less stressful than it might have been, despite my goal-kicking anxieties.

FIVE

STORMING THE FORTRESS

I'VE OFTEN THOUGHT THAT part of the reason the loss at Eden Park in 1991 was so disappointing was that we'd won there in 1986 in not dissimilar conditions. It's just such an incredibly tough place to win. The term 'fortress' is one that you hear used a lot to describe grounds that are hard places to win at. Sometimes it's misused, exaggerated. But Eden Park really is a fortress. It's not just Australia that struggles to win there. Everyone finds it hard.

I remember Alan Jones and I exchanging emails about that very subject in July 2014 when we were discussing Australia's chances of winning the Eden Park Test a month later. Jonesy said, 'Is this the year?' There was at least reason for optimism. Australia had held the All Blacks to a competitive 12–12 draw in Sydney the week previously. It didn't seem implausible.

I told Alan that I had mixed feelings. There was part of me that wanted the Wallabies to win. I want Australia to win *every*

Test they play. That's the proud patriot in me. But there's another side of me that hopes they never win at Eden Park again, just so our win in 1986 remains in the record books as the last time Australia prevailed there. It's a nice result to be associated with.

I needn't have worried. As it turned out, Australia were run over 51–20. I was very disappointed, but in a strange way I was also relieved.

In addition to the fact that we won a series in New Zealand in 1986, my other enduring memory of that tour is the same one that I can recall about every trip to New Zealand: it's always extremely tough. There were lots of matches—Saturday and then Wednesday—and it didn't matter if you were playing the All Blacks or Manawatu; it was bloody hard. Every single game was a tough physical contest. But if you come out of it all and win a Test series, it's probably one of the most rewarding things you can do as a rugby player. It's the All Blacks, after all, that you're playing, and that's who you measure yourself against.

But New Zealand is a country of contrasts. Off the field, people couldn't be more hospitable and helpful. We Aussies were treated like royalty—rugby is the absolute number-one sport in the entire country. If you wanted to go fishing, wanted to go on a jet-boat trip or play golf, it was there on a platter for you. The locals were kind and treated you very well; then on the pitch you were absolutely blasted. That's how it always was. But we responded to that by training harder than ever before on that tour, and it paid off when we won the first Test in Wellington.

I never had vendettas against rugby grounds per se, but Athletic Park in Wellington and I never got along. I always hated playing in Wellington. It was always windy. There was a huge stand on one side and a smaller one on the other, with absolutely nothing at either end. The wind howled down the ground all day every day; it was like a huge funnel.

We played against a team that was nicknamed the 'Baby Blacks' that day. Because of the New Zealand Cavaliers' rebel tour to South Africa earlier that year, some of the regular All Blacks had been suspended for two Tests as a punishment—the first was against Scotland and the second was the Test against us in Wellington. Some of those suspended players struggled to regain or retain their places after the ban. It was quite a controversial period in world rugby.

As usual, there was probably a forty-knot wind blowing down the ground in Wellington that day and it made rugby very difficult. Surprisingly, playing against the wind wasn't such a huge problem. But playing with the wind was almost impossible because your halfback would be passing *into* the wind to get it to you. As a result, the ball would float—often for long enough for an All Black flanker to arrive at the same time. It was a flyhalf's nightmare from every perspective. It was really hard to play any kind of constructive rugby in those conditions. Nick was fantastic in these kinds of situations, though. He knew how to keep the ball close by going up the blindside in short little snipes then back inside to the forwards; he was absolutely terrific. It was a very physical game but we did enough to take it 13–12.

NICK FARR-JONES, FORMER WALLABY HALFBACK: I loved having Michael outside me because he took so much pressure off me. He was the decision-maker and 99 per cent of the time his decision-making was spot on. I always knew exactly where he'd be; I always heard his voice clearly. We had very good empathy towards each other on the field.

The second Test down in Dunedin two weeks later is one we should have won. But we never won in Dunedin; I've never been entirely sure why. It's just one of those grounds where things always seemed to go against us. But we thought we'd done enough to win when Steve Tuynman went over for a try with just a few minutes left, only for the referee, Derek Bevan, to disallow it.

We never knew why. Apparently he never knew why either. It was a try, no doubt about it. And in the after-match reception Bevan said to us, 'Sorry guys, I got that one wrong. It *was* a try.' It was big of him to admit the error, but I thought, 'Great, but your mistake might cost us the Bledisloe Cup.' It was bitterly disappointing. Alan Jones still talks about it now.

Unbeknownst to us at the time, if we'd won in Dunedin and lifted the Bledisloe Cup with it, we would have had three days of relaxation to look forward to down in Queenstown—a resort town in Otago. Instead, we had to go to Invercargill on the Sunday to prepare for a midweek game against Southland. None of us was particularly excited about that prospect. We drove most of the day from Dunedin and arrived in Invercargill on the Sunday night. Everybody was disappointed, really down, and Alan Jones was calling the Test team into his room one by one while we were sitting in the bar having a drink.

One by one the guys came out saying, 'We've got the day off tomorrow—Jonesy's given us the day off.' So Slacky comes out next—'Mate, I've got the day off too. After you've been in, we'll organise a golf game for the morning.' I thought, 'That's great.'

When my turn came to go into the room, Alan said, 'Michael, I've got some great news for you.' I was thinking, 'Fantastic, here we go, golf, terrific!' but then he said, 'Southland: really tough team. But I'm going to make you captain and fullback.' I said, 'What? Captain and fullback?' and he said, 'Yeah, you deserve to captain your country—what a great honour.'

I agreed. 'That's great. What an honour.' But what I actually thought was, 'Shit, I've never played fullback and here I am playing against Southland where all they do is kick it up in the air, run through and bash whoever catches it.'

Out I come from the room and Slacky and a few others are there going, 'So mate, what time are we going to play golf?' and I said, 'Mate, I'm off to training tomorrow. He's made me captain and fullback.'

So off I went to training the next morning while all the other Test players were taking it easy. It was funny, because we were doing all these new moves with a revamped back line. Normally the fullback is the guy who injects from wide and behind—adds the pace, coming in at an angle and all that kind of thing. But because I was so slow and tired, I literally had to start in front of my outside centre to chime into the back line at all. I wasn't injecting any pace whatsoever. I was just trying to keep up with them.

Anyway, Invercargill was pretty wet and windy, as usual, with Southland out to get us—to take a big Australian scalp and make a bit of a name for themselves. But we got through the game, won it and moved on to the final Test at Eden Park.

In that third Test, the All Blacks really surprised us. They picked a big physical pack of forwards and we assumed they'd try to soften us up. But instead they came out running the ball from everywhere. Frano Botica, a running five-eighth, was at ten that day and they really caught us off guard for a while. As soon as the whistle blew, away they went. But eventually we clawed our way back into the game.

I remember a penalty we got in the second half. It was a pretty long way out and it was slippery underfoot, with the cricket pitch in the middle making it worse. I looked at it, noted the dodgy surface conditions, and said to Slacky, 'I'll have a go.'

It was a tough kick, but I got it. Very rarely do I show any kind of emotion on the pitch, but this time I allowed myself a little air punch on the way back. It was a hugely important moment and it just about took us beyond their reach. Then Campo scored a try and that was it. We'd won and we'd won well. Mission accomplished. It was a massively satisfying achievement.

As for the 'fortress' Eden Park hoodoo, I've thought about it many times over the years. Alan Jones has been quoted as saying that it's nothing to do with the ground and everything to do with teams not being good enough. Some would argue that, given that he coached the 1986 team, he would say that. Even if that were true, you'd think by the law of averages that an Australian team would win there *sometime*—'Every time you lose one, you're closer to the one you're going to win', as the saying goes. But that sometime never seems to arrive.

But, as I said, it's not just Australia that hasn't won there. Everybody struggles there and of course the All Blacks use that to their advantage. *They* believe in Eden Park's aura—'This is our place—go away!' Every All Black team now feels like they are defending the honour there. Nobody wants to be part of the team that loses at Eden Park after thirty years.

But when you boil it all down and remove the myth, Eden Park, like every other ground, is just a piece of grass. They're all the same size nowadays too. They've all got lines in the same places. It shouldn't be an issue. Admittedly, back in those days, before it was redeveloped, Eden Park was quite oddly shaped. The stands didn't sit parallel to the sideline and the ends didn't sit square with the deadball area. It was an awkward ground and the wind used to swirl around all over the place.

Carisbrook in Dunedin was the same—it was a cricket ground too. Australia has only ever won once there, and that was as recently as 2001. That's an even more amazing statistic when you think about it. Eden Park is always called the fortress, but Dunedin is every bit as difficult a place to win, perhaps even more.

SIX

THE BAD OLD DAYS

DRESSING ROOMS CAN BE fantastic places when you win. Everyone always said that Eden Park's dressing room, down in the concrete bowels, was a scary place because you could hear all the noise above you. After we won there it wasn't scary. All the noise was ours.

Everyone was smiling, drinking champagne from the Bledisloe Cup as if it was All Black blood; Slacky wearing an All Black jersey while doing so ... these are the highs, and you savour the taste of them because soon they are gone.

The flipside is that a dressing room can be a pretty grim place after a defeat. On *this* occasion, in 1987, you could literally hear a pin drop. I just stared at an imaginary spot on the wall, above and to the left of Brett Papworth's head. I couldn't think what else to do.

After twenty minutes our coach, Alan Jones, said, 'Jeez, would somebody turn the damn showers on. It's far too quiet in here.' At least he'd broken the ice. A few of us started talking, discussing what had happened out there. How they'd won it. How we'd lost it.

One of the questions I've been asked most often is whether losing to France in the semi-final of the 1987 World Cup was the most disappointing moment of my career. It wasn't. I remember thinking a few times: 'No, it's the *second* most disappointing moment.' It was beaten soundly by the precise moment in the Concord Oval dressing room when, as we desperately analysed how we'd let the semi-final slip, our manager John Breen came in and told us that we had to leave early the next morning to go to Rotorua to play Wales in the third-place playoff. For some reason that actually hurt more.

'Be down in the foyer, bags packed and ready to leave at 7am.'

It was devastating news. We hadn't even considered the third-place playoff. All we'd been thinking was, 'Let's win this and get to the World Cup Final.' Having to pick ourselves up and get motivated for what seemed like a meaningless match did not appeal much.

'Who cares who comes third?' was followed closely by, 'Is there no way to get out of this?'

There was no way out—we had to play.

The run-up to the 1987 World Cup was quite strange, on reflection. We obviously knew that it was a pretty big deal because the press was building it up. But at the same time— given that it was the first World Cup—it was a complete unknown. Nobody had anything to compare it to.

Because a lot of our pool games were in Sydney, the guys who lived there, like Nick Farr-Jones and Simon Poidevin, went to work in the morning as usual and turned up to training in the afternoon in their own cars—business as usual.

For us Queenslanders, though—guys like me, Slacky, Andy McIntyre, Bill Campbell and Anthony Herbert—it was as if we were on an overseas tour. There was an immediate imbalance. Even our coach, Jones, was continuing with his morning radio show at 2UE, so we never saw him in the team hotel until around lunchtime—not that many of us were up by then because, during the evenings, we'd head out on the town.

We'd be sitting around the lobby like a bunch of university students. Except we were a bunch of unsupervised amateur rugby players.

'Okay, where are we going tonight, boys?'

'Anyone hungry?'

'Let's go and get some pizza.'

'How about that Italian restaurant round the corner?'

So three or four of us might do that, or go to the pub, or go and see a band somewhere. I remember that Died Pretty—a really good pub-rock band that released a load of albums in the '80s and '90s—was in residence at a bar just round the corner from the hotel. I went and saw them twice and had a couple of beers. It was great. But it didn't feel like a World Cup build-up.

Guys would sleep in until eleven o'clock or midday pretty regularly, get up for training and then go out at night. We didn't stay out ridiculously late, say until 4am. Some nights we stayed out latish, though. It wasn't an intentionally lazy routine; it's just how the days worked out. Our body clocks had been moved back a few hours because we knew we didn't need to get started early in the mornings.

It was never full-on debauchery, but it wasn't the optimum physical preparation and nothing like a World Cup build-up of the twenty-first century. We simply knew that we didn't ever have to train until the afternoon.

The result was a subtle divide in the camp, a slight lack of unity. Nothing major, but it was there. We Queenslanders felt isolated when we were in Sydney—as I'm sure the other guys did when we played in Brisbane. I'm not suggesting that this imbalance created any animosity among the squad—not at all. I'm pretty sure the New South Wales guys would have done exactly the same thing if we'd been based in Brisbane for the majority of the tournament. But it didn't create the ideal environment to prepare for what was a World Championship event, albeit a very amateur one in those days. We all knew each other pretty well, but we weren't as tight-knit a group as we probably could have been—maybe that's the best way of summing it up.

As far as the tournament went, it was pretty obvious to most people that New Zealand were the favourites. Of all the other teams, we were the one considered most likely to beat them, and our pool draw with England, Japan and the USA made progression look reasonably straightforward. Worryingly, it seemed as if some of the more lethargic aspects of our preparation had been transported onto the playing field when we went behind to a Mike Harrison try in our opening pool game against England at Concord Oval. It felt like a few of us were still in the pub.

Tries from Campo and Poidevin and a few kicks from me got us back in the game and in the end we came out 19–6 winners. We certainly weren't at our best, but we hadn't needed to be. We did enough.

Relatively easy wins in our other two pool games booked us a quarter-final appointment with Ireland in Sydney on June 7th and, theoretically, ensured that we would avoid New Zealand until the final in Auckland. We beat Ireland fairly comfortably in Sydney and then only France stood between us and the first-ever World Cup final.

My good friend Philippe Sella always says that the semi-final between France and Australia in Sydney on June 13th 1987 is the greatest Test match he ever played in. Philippe ended up being capped 111 times for France so he's pretty well qualified to judge. Many people have described it as one of the greatest Test matches ever played.

Me? Even though we lost it, I would probably agree.

It was such a great game of rugby. It was close, the lead changed constantly; you just never quite knew what was going to happen until that Blanco try at the end. But at no point did I ever feel, 'I'm part of history here.' You don't have the time to register the significance. It was purely a game of rugby and it was my job to work out a way to win it.

Speaking of that last-minute try, I've watched it a few times recently and it looks a little suspect. We have TMOs (video referees) nowadays and I reckon that try might have been disallowed if they'd had that technology back then. If I was the referee I'd definitely be saying, 'Let's have a look ...'

The bloke who tackled Serge Blanco in the corner was our seventeen- stone hooker, Tommy Lawton. How he got there I'll never know, and, remember, back in 1987 the corner flag was considered to be 'out'. Tommy definitely had most of Blanco in touch before the ball went down. And I don't just say that because of a mistake I made in the lead-up to the try.

On the third or fourth phase of an intense passage of French possession, there was half a chance of an interception. Patrice Lagisquet's inside pass looped up in the air for what seemed an eternity. Instinctively I went for the ball because I thought it was there to be had, but Eric Champ arrived at the same time and snapped it out of my hands. The way I snatched at the ball doesn't look too good when I watch the footage. But had I taken the ball, we would have had a good chance of scoring down the other end. It was one of those instinctive decisions that you make in a split second. It could have worked in our favour. It didn't. It gifted France the game.

The ball bounced backwards towards their number eight, Laurent Rodriguez, who, as he scooped it up before slinging the match-winning pass to Blanco, knocked it on. It was a tiny movement in a very frenetic period of play. If you watch the footage, it's barely noticeable. But the ball did go forward and we paused for a split second expecting the whistle to blow. Later replays confirmed the knock-on, but the referee didn't call it at the time. It was just one of those things—an example of the fine line between winning and losing.

ALAN JONES, FORMER AUSTRALIAN COACH: Rodriguez's knock-on still haunts me. Michael was in possession shortly beforehand and I always remember wishing that he'd kicked it up the other end of the field. As it turned out, we almost stopped playing when the knock-on occurred but the referee didn't pick up on it, they scored in the corner and converted it. In all honesty, it was a game that we shouldn't have lost.

Earlier in the game I experienced one of the more surreal moments of my entire career, let alone this match. My dummy to wrong-foot Franck Mesnel and a step inside Philippe Sella set up a break deep inside French territory. As he usually did, Campo showed up at the end of the move to score in the corner after Peter Grigg popped the ball inside to him. It was a try that gave him the Australian record for try-scoring at that time. It also left me with a conversion from the right-hand touchline, right in front of the grandstand. In the context of the match, it was a vital kick and would give us a slender three-point lead with only fifteen minutes left.

Back in 1987, we were still using a few handfuls of loose sand as a platform for the ball, as plastic tees had yet to be invented. So the ball boy came onto the field with the little bucket of sand and it was part of my routine, as I was preparing my sand tee, to look up and say 'Thank you'. It was something I always did. I thought it was a nice thing to do. But as I was putting the ball down, I was aware of this ball boy—probably twelve years old—still standing there. I looked up at him as if to say, 'You shouldn't still be here.'

He didn't move.

'This is a pretty important kick, mate ...'

I couldn't believe what I was hearing. It was a bizarre moment of personal interaction in the midst of a momentous occasion. But for a moment it was as if he and I were the only two left at Concord Oval.

'Thanks, I know.' I said. 'This is the semi-final of the World Cup.'

'Well, you better get it,' he said, before trotting off.

I did get it and as I was running back for the restart, I glanced over and saw him standing on the touchline giving me the thumbs-up with a big smile on his face. I'll never forget it.

When I review the game in detail, it's clear to me that I made another important mistake. Why is it the mistakes that you remember best? I missed a tackle to allow Philippe Sella to score under the posts early in the second half. Philippe was very strong and highly evasive—a really *hard* runner. In addition to that—and I only really found this out many years later when he and I played together at Saracens—the French didn't have much of a structured game plan to implement. Whereas we had pre-determined, sometimes intricate moves designed to get across the gain line, create defensive confusion and then score tries, the French just *ran*. Their policy was pretty simple: get deep, pass the ball—shimmy a little bit here and *run* ... Then Serge Blanco would get involved and anything could happen. It was all so free and easy—so French.

Saying all that, Australia had quite a good defensive pattern, certainly for defending set pieces, which in those days were considered to be the best positions from which to attack. But once play broke up or a kick went up and the ball started bouncing here and there, our defensive pattern went out the window and it became a case of all hands on deck. Consequently, I ended up covering a lot. Hence, in both the Blanco try and the Sella one earlier, I ended up pretty close to the person who scored.

In Philippe's case, I was coming across in cover and he just stepped inside me. I was so nervous about being on my own on the outside that I left him the inside, which he gratefully accepted. There was very little I could have done about it other than stick out a hopeful arm as he went past (which I tried).

As tough as it was to accept, France did to us what they often seemed to manage in later World Cups: they found a great performance from practically nowhere—one that didn't correlate with their previous form. They pulled a result out of thin air. Because of the way they played and the talented players they had in key positions, there was always that potential to turn a game on its head.

In fairness to them, in front of all the flair and unpredictability in the back line, their forwards were extremely tough. I remember the first lineout of the semi-final clearly. It set a precedent. Eric Champ, who was a big guy for the time and a pretty crazy-looking character to go with it, took a step away from the lineout and stared directly at me, muttering and pointing towards me with a look on his face that said, 'Lynagh, I'm coming for you. I'm going to kill you.' My French wasn't good enough to get his exact meaning, but I'm in no doubt it was something along those lines.

Never having been a fan of the actual physical contact part of the game, I remember thinking, 'Oh *shit* …' while taking a couple of backward steps, not, 'All right Eric, let's have some fun.'

NICK FARR-JONES: One of Michael's great strengths was that he always stayed out of the deep, dark places—the combat zone. It's a very good skill to have and that comes down to his decision-making. I hardly ever saw Michael getting shoed by anybody; he always seemed to stay out of it.

I did three full tours of France. The first and most memorable was in 1983. Despite the devastating World Cup loss, I always enjoyed playing against the French. France tested teams in different ways: by being very physical, running the ball, kicking it; the overall standard was always very high. They were always hard.

Were they dirty? Probably. Not all of them, but most of the forwards tried to intimidate you. I remember the first game of the '83 tour; it was up in Strasbourg. They just belted us. The first lineout was a full-on brawl. They wanted to soften us up and I'm glad I was on the bench. Steve Tuynman almost had his ear ripped off. He was young, like I was. I remember looking at it in the dressing room afterwards; you could actually see cartilage. It was brutal. But you just had to get on with it.

Also on that '83 tour, there was some pretty dubious refereeing. I remember one occasion when I kicked a drop goal. There was no question about it. We'd all started running back. But the referee just went, 'Non—no goal. Twenty-two.' Our captain, Slacky, just couldn't believe it.

But when I run into the French guys now, I always get on very well with them. Even the forwards, who tried to kill us back then. Nowadays, they are friendly and open. They'll have dinner with you, have a beer with you—they're very hospitable and always treat you well. I only wish I could speak better French.

Even though I haven't seen him for a few years, Jean-Pierre Rives is someone I've always got on very well with. He's an interesting guy. He's a renowned painter and sculptor; he exhibits his work all over the world. Blanco was an interesting character too. He smoked a lot—that was common knowledge. In recent years, I've occasionally run into him in Biarritz, where he lives. We go down there on holiday a couple of times a year. He doesn't speak much English. Or at least he pretends he doesn't. He's as enigmatic as he ever was, but what a great player.

All the French players I run into are nice, friendly guys who've moved on, as I have, since retiring from the game. The great thing about rugby is that, whenever you all meet, there's that common bond that holds you together. I really think that the sport is unique in that way—perhaps more so than other team sports.

AFTER THE DISAPPOINTMENT OF Sydney, the third-place playoff in Rotorua was a mere footnote. It didn't help that David Codey got himself sent off in the first five minutes, somewhat unfairly in retrospect, for trampling in a couple of the rucks.

We spent most of the game with fourteen men on the field. Ultimately, we lost 21–22 with a last-minute conversion from the touchline by Paul Thorburn. It was so disappointing, but an appropriate cherry on the cake of the defeat in Sydney. The record books say that we were the fourth-best team in the competition, but I'm not sure how many people would agree with that.

SEVEN

FOUR MINUTES
OF MAGIC

GRANT FOX: While I'm sure Michael was affected by the missed kick at Eden Park, I've always been of the opinion that that defeat in Auckland was what helped them win the World Cup. It was the most important game in Australia's 1991 World Cup victory, apart from the actual games at the tournament itself.

THE EMOTIONAL SCARS THAT Eden Park in 1991 had left on my psyche were always with me. They were like stubborn stains on my rugby brain and I felt that the only way of erasing them was to stand in front of the next important kick as soon as possible. But as a team we were pretty confident about the 1991 World Cup going into it. Losing to the All Blacks, regardless of how it had happened, had done us a favour, it seemed. The Australian press weren't hyping us; nobody else was either. We thought, 'Maybe we can fly under the radar a little here.' The All Blacks, on the other hand, were all the rage.

There was no doubting our team was a good one. Several of us, probably myself included, were at or approaching the peaks of our careers. We were also pretty relaxed and unburdened. Although we'd lost the Bledisloe Cup, we'd played well enough against a touring Welsh side and then, later, a very good England side in a Sydney Test match in July, suggesting we'd definitely be in the mix in the latter stages of the competition.

BOB DWYER: We were the best team going into the 1991 World Cup. There was absolutely no doubt about that. We'd given England a hell of a hiding and were more than New Zealand's equal. We were also smart enough to know that none of that mattered. It was all about what we did each day. That was our focus.

The 1991 World Cup is memorable for me for several reasons. Everyone talks about the Ireland game, the quarter-final—that try in the last minute that dug us out of a hole. Or rather, a chasm. But apart from actually lifting the Webb Ellis trophy at Twickenham, that's not the memory that sticks with me most. Lansdowne Road was fabulous, yes, but it was four minutes of magic. And there were still two more bridges to cross after it. In the background of all of this, I was still really struggling with my goal-kicking.

We were using the same ball we'd used in Auckland and I seemed unable to break the cycle of doubt and anxiety, despite adjusting my preparation by changing my pre-kick approach. That missed kick was still on my mind. No matter how much I practised to perfect my execution, it was always in my head, going, 'Remember me?' every time I stood in front of a kick.

In an attempt to iron out the problems and restore my shattered confidence, I practised more than I ever had previously. I used to stand at the corner flag in practice and kick along the goal line. The point was to hit the post; the aim was just to use a line that someone had conveniently put there to focus on kicking the ball down a particular path. In a way I was taking some of the pressure off myself by removing the conventional goalposts from the equation. It seemed to help when I came to actually aim between the posts in matches.

Despite that, I still had a lot of trouble with conversions or penalties that were ten metres either side of the posts. Maybe it was because these are the kicks you should get, the ones everyone expects you to get. I'm sure I was overthinking them—'What am I going to do here?' It was really unsettling me, not that you'd have known if you looked at the bare results.

On paper, I was successful in the pool games against Argentina, Wales and Samoa. I think I kicked seven penalties and seven conversions. I don't know what the percentages were, but hey, that was still fourteen successes. But believe me, every time I stepped up to a kick, I had this mental dialogue going back and forth in my head as my practical brain tried to overcome my confidence's cautionary warnings.

'I want to kick from really close to the posts.' That would make it harder to miss.

'But wait! If I do that, I'm increasing the chances of having the kick charged down.'

'Let's shorten my run-up to avoid that.'

'Fine, but at what stage when you go out wider do you revert to your old run-up?'

TIM HORAN, FORMER WALLABY CENTRE: I remember Noddy having problems in England. Whenever he practised, he did this strange thing where he never lined up directly in front. Instead, he aimed at one post—almost as if he wanted to take the actual getting the ball between the posts out of the equation.

On and on it went. All these insecurities and peripheral questions were in my head during every game. I tried to fix it in the practice sessions by getting the guys to run at me to simulate charge-downs. I kicked goals from every conceivable place in every pitch before each match. I lay in bed every night before games, rehearsing every kick I could possibly be presented with the next day. On the surface, and on paper, I was getting through the World Cup. But in my mind it was as big a challenge as it had ever been. Every kick was a battle. The demons just wouldn't leave me.

IAN LYNAGH: I was over in the UK with Michael and I even went out on the training pitch with him one day to try and help. He was spraying even the simplest kicks because he was really caught up in his own head. To me, that was indicative of the huge trauma he'd gone through when missing that kick in Auckland. His confidence was blown apart. Michael can be a bit obsessive in terms of detail sometimes and I believe that he was overthinking everything during the World Cup in 1991.

It was no consolation to me to consider that I probably wasn't alone in having these problems. I was only concerned with what *I* was doing. In any case, it wasn't the kind of thing you discussed with other goal-kickers. There's an unspoken rule that you don't admit to your problems, certainly not while you're still playing.

GRANT FOX: I understand Michael's mental anguish. It's a little bit like John Kirwan [former All Black winger] talking about depression. I played a lot of rugby with JK and he never shared it, nor did I notice it. It's only now, all these years later, that he comes out with what he was going through. Michael's problems with goal-kicking were never obvious to me. I never even sensed it. Having heard it, I now understand it. Nowadays, whenever I'm asked to coach youngsters, the first question I ask is: 'Do you want to be the goal-kicker? Do you want to stand in front of 50,000 people and the millions watching on television? If you don't relish that attention and can't cope with what comes with it, best you leave now.' But it was only once I stopped playing that I began to think about it in those terms.

With hindsight, it occurred to me that my reluctance to disclose or discuss my problems was like the attitude of a golfer who has just come off the course after a bad round. They'll never actually *say* they played badly. That would be counter-productive and would undermine what little remaining positivity they have left. 'I missed a few putts today but I'll go away and work on it—we'll be okay. I'm in a good place,' is what they say, not, 'I'm playing badly and I've no idea what to do about it.' They always keep it positive. It's as if by saying these things, it somehow makes them true. The same applies to goal-kickers: they'll never admit they're struggling.

I WAS RECENTLY REMINDED of how I used to feel. I was watching an international with my eldest son. It was an autumn Saturday in 2013. The goal-kicker for one side was lining up a last-minute penalty that would have given his team a pretty significant win. It wouldn't be fair of me to name names and it doesn't actually matter; it's just an example. It wasn't, in the scheme of things, a difficult kick: it was ten or fifteen metres wide of the right-hand post—the kind of kick that should be considered routine, even in a high-pressure situation, as this was. Just as the goal-kicker drew breath and settled for a few seconds longer than you might expect at the beginning of his run-up, my son turned to me and said, 'I reckon he's going to miss this.' I was interested in his intuition. 'What makes you say that?'

'Oh, he's just taking too long. He's worried.'

'Mate,' I said, 'that's really perceptive of you. You are absolutely right.'

And of course he did miss the kick and I think he's had a problem with kicks like that since then—not that he'd ever dream of admitting it.

As an international goal-kicker in the modern game, unless you're kicking 85 per cent plus, you're not really delivering. The stadiums nowadays are enclosed, the pitches are perfect and players practise all day, every day. Everything's in your favour.

But you've still got to put the ball down and kick it…

In recent years, Jonny Wilkinson has been responsible for taking goal-kicking to the incredible level it is currently at. I don't know Jonny very well. I'm not sure if anyone really does. He's a complete one-off. But none of the top guys miss much nowadays because Jonny showed them how not to. And a lot of that is due to his incredible work ethic. Jonny has taken that part of the game to new levels also. But I'm sure he'd give a lot of credit to his kicking coach, Dave Aldred, who also coached the golfer Luke Donald. I'm guessing that Aldred kept Jonny focused less on overthinking and more on the act of striking the ball. Even so, I'd be surprised if even Jonny hadn't had days when he thought, 'Oh no, I don't want to have to kick this.' We've all had those days.

GRANT FOX: Sometimes I didn't want the opportunity. I'd sometimes think, 'Don't give us a penalty. I don't want to step up.' I can't recall specific instances when it happened, but I'm not denying that it happened. Generally, when I missed one in my early days, I thought, 'I want to get back on the horse quickly.' I got pissed off for missing and wanted another opportunity. In my mid-career, my expectations became unrealistic and that's when the doubt set in—'I don't want the opportunity.' Then you learn to isolate everything kick by kick, reconciling the years of practice. A bad kick is just a bad kick. You isolate it. For the next kick, you focus on the process, not the negative thoughts. Trust that you know how to do it—trust the mechanics. But it's hard to get to that point when you can separate the mental and the physical process.

When you think about it, the similarities between swinging a golf club and kicking a rugby ball are remarkable. They are both stationary objects. And if you substitute the kicking leg for a golf club, the rest comes down to repeating the same routine and mechanics time after time—grooving yourself to repeat the same movement, regardless of conditions. The only difference is that the golfers get paid a little more for doing it.

I remember that on more than a few occasions before big games my dad would take me down to the driving range just to loosen me up by hitting a few golf balls. It was helpful on a couple of levels. First, it took me away from that awful sitting about, feeling physically sick with nerves about goal-kicking. Secondly, it was all about going through the ball towards your target. Dad really understood that connection.

But in golf, when you're lining up a twenty-foot putt or hitting a tee shot into a par three, nobody's been tackling you and wrestling you to the ground for the few minutes prior to that. Golfers are able to stay in the same calm mode, but rugby players in the midst of a full-contact situation simply can't.

This golf–rugby analogy was reinforced for me when I played in the 2005 Wales Open golf pro-am at Celtic Manor with Michael Campbell from New Zealand. He was playing beautifully that day and made a few excellent putts. But he'd had a pretty shocking year to that point. On the way from one of the greens to the next tee I chatted to his caddie: 'Why is he having such a poor year? He's hitting the ball great.'

'He's starting to get there … it's coming,' the caddie said, with a bit of a knowing gleam in his eye.

When we reached the par three 13th hole there were a couple of groups waiting to play in front of us. Michael—a big rugby fan—and I sat down on a bench together and he struck up a non-golf-related conversation.

'So …' he said, 'did you ever have any problems with your goal-kicking?'

'Definitely, mate,' I said, and because we had a bit of a wait until we were up on the tee, I had plenty of time to tell him a story about the 1984 Wallaby tour to the UK—the Grand Slam Tour.

I was the kicker. I was playing centre; Mark Ella was at ten.

I didn't kick well against England. Didn't kick well against Ireland. I was dropped for the goal-kicking against Wales; Roger Gould took over and kicked everything. *Everything.* I scored a try. We won the game and even then I was thinking, 'Jeez, I might not get this job back.'

ALAN JONES: The publicity surrounding this Australian team just kept building and building. There was a lot of pressure on them. Michael was starting to get a bit wayward with his kicking after the Ireland game so I thought I'd give him a rest from it all. We were on a visit to the Waterford Crystal factory in Ireland and I called him out. 'Look, you've had a really hard tour—a lot of pressure. I'm going to take the pressure away from you. I'm taking you off the goal-kicking.' Straight away, this serious little face looked at me and said, 'Are you dropping me?' 'Will you wake up?' I said. 'Of course I'm not dropping you. You'll be in the Test against Wales; I just don't want you to kick goals.' He didn't even ask who was going to kick goals—he was as happy as a pig in mud.

We arrived in Scotland for the Grand Slam decider. Alan Jones couldn't decide who the kicker was going to be. Me, who couldn't kick a goal in the matches, or Roger Gould, who couldn't miss one. It was pretty obvious, you'd think.

IAN LYNAGH: Kicking is not an intellectual thing. It's a psycho-motor action. So the more you can keep your head out of it, the better you'll do. You've got to trust the feeling. The problem was that Alan Jones's way is to intellectualise everything. He'd stand next to Michael when he was practising and that wasn't helping, although

Alan was genuinely trying to help. Michael rang me a few times on that trip, worried about what was happening. 'You're getting too much input, first of all,' I told him. Then I made him a relaxation tape and sent it over. I also had a few other ideas to do with the position he was playing.

I'd been talking to Dad on the phone during that week—'At training I can't miss, but in the games they're just missing.'

And soon he'd worked out why. It was because I was playing centre as opposed to flyhalf. During the midweek games I'd been playing flyhalf and kicking everything. But when I went to centre to play outside Mark Ella, which in those days was a much more confrontational, defensive position than flyhalf, my kicking was influenced by the fact that I was playing at a much higher arousal level physically. So when I came to do the goal-kicking, my heart rate was up—everything was at high intensity and functioning that bit quicker. As a result, the kicks were just off. Not much, but enough. At training, you're not in the same elevated state. I thought, 'That's genius.'

One day at training before the Scotland game, Roger and I had a kick-off. Alan Jones was watching. I couldn't miss; Roger couldn't miss. Jonesy ended up calling me into his room on the Saturday morning to give me the goal-kicking duties. He said, 'You'll be kicking today—I trust you.' It was a very tough call that he made. I think he thought that his brilliant management of me was the key. He *had* handled it well; he always did. He was massively intelligent. He understood people, me included. But the real reason was that Dad had discovered what had been causing me the problems.

NICK FARR-JONES: Alan Jones's main strength was knowing how to handle people. I remember him giving me a pretty solid kick up the arse on that tour and that was precisely what I needed. He perceived me as being a guy who just went on tour to have fun. That was true, but I also prepared and worked my arse off. With Michael, Jones knew how to handle his sensitivities. Michael and I were great friends, but very different people. Jones recognised that difference.

Dad had given me something to think about, and then he came up with a great suggestion. 'When there's a penalty or conversion, what I want you to do is press, subconsciously, a slow-motion button.' His theory applied to everything that happened after the whistle was blown for a penalty or in the preparation for a conversion attempt. Breathing, walking, talking, fixing the ball, interacting with the ball boy—everything was to be done in slow motion.

I practised the slow-motion technique and then when I went out for the game at Murrayfield, I slotted the first one over from way out on the left touchline. It went right down the middle. Beautiful. I then kicked an Australian record, pressing the slow-motion button every time.

So I told Michael Campbell all this. 'Wow, that's fantastic,' he said. We went on to finish in the top five as a team and he finished fourth in the whole event.

Afterwards, we had a few beers. I asked him what was next.

'I've got to go to the US Open Qualifier at Walton Heath on Monday, with about a hundred others.'

Because he hadn't been playing well, he didn't even want to go. He thought he had no chance. But his caddie had talked him into it—'Come on mate, what have we got to lose?'

He qualified. *Just.* Got into the US Open at Pinehurst. Next thing you know he was posting a last-day 69 to hold off Tiger Woods by two shots and win. After he hit his tee shot on the eighteenth into the rough and hacked it out into the fairway, he left the course for a toilet break. Then he came back to play the most important shot of his life: a chip over a bunker that he knocked close to the hole. He'd had a similar shot at Walton Heath to qualify in the first place. On both occasions, he holed the putts.

I texted him straight afterwards to say congratulations and four or five days later he got back to me.

'Mate, thanks very much. I pressed the slow-motion button on the eighteenth.'

He'd followed my advice. It worked for him, or so he told me.

THE LEAST IMPORTANT MOMENT of the 1991 World Cup quarter-final against Ireland was the conversion attempt I had with seconds winding down. Given how I was feeling about goal-kicking, it was quite refreshing that I didn't have to get it. And I didn't get it. But we'd all but won the game anyway.

Sir Clive Woodward, the England coach, had a concept called TCUP that he used with his World Cup winning team in 2003. It stands for 'Thinking Clearly Under Pressure'. Someone once told me that Woodward held up my decision-making during the last five minutes of the 1991 World Cup quarter-final in Dublin as being the best possible example of it in sport. That's a massive compliment. It was certainly a very significant passage of play for me, for a number of reasons, least of all that I scored the winning try.

We were pretty heavy favourites to beat Ireland. Nick Farr-Jones, our captain, had to be substituted very early through injury, and I was given the captain's armband. We always felt we were in control. But you've still got to put teams away. We had most of the play—we even had a couple of tries disallowed for forward passes—but whenever we looked up at the scoreboard, Ireland were still there, lurking just behind us. We couldn't seem to pull away from them and put the game beyond doubt.

An enduring memory for me, as goal-kicker, was how incredibly quiet the stadium was whenever I prepared to kick. When you're playing suburban club rugby in Brisbane, for example, there might only be four hundred people there. But they'd be only a metre away. You'd hear every little comment and there was always somebody saying something—'Jeez, this is a hard kick, mate. I don't think you're going to get this.' That didn't get to me at all. But in Dublin, the deathly silence unnerved me because it reminded me not only that I was kicking for vital points, but also that sixty thousand people were there at the ground and were all intently watching *me*.

We kept nudging ahead in the game, doing just enough, until a little mistake somewhere in defence when we were recovering a kick-through allowed the Irish flanker Gordon Hamilton to go over in the corner with four minutes left. Even as a player on the opposing side, I couldn't help but register the potential romance of the situation. It was absolute mayhem. Lansdowne Road went berserk. Ireland led us 16–15. There was literally a pitch invasion. Before Ralph Keyes kicked the conversion from the sideline to make it 18–15, I thought, 'Okay, I'm the captain. What are we going to do?'

My next thought was, 'Let's deal in certainties.' So I went to the referee, Jim Fleming, and asked him how long there was to go. He said, 'Four minutes.' When I got back to the goal line the guys were standing there, heads down, going, 'We're gone.'

I disagreed. I thought, 'There's time.' I didn't want to deal in negatives. How often do you hear people use the word 'don't' in a tense situation? 'Don't do this; don't panic; don't worry.' It's not a good word. So instead I said to the guys, 'We've got four minutes; this is what we're going to *do*.'

I decided that we'd kick off long and then they'd kick for touch and that would give us a lineout in their half. We'd win the ball and then we, the backs, would look after it from there. I knew the outcome I wanted. I set small step-by-step goals. I said, 'If you end up with the ball and are in any doubt, hold on to it and just keep going forward.'

We kicked off long and their halfback, Rob Saunders, sliced his kick badly. We ended up with a lineout inside their twenty-two. We were already ahead of the game plan.

We'd done a move, called 'S', a few times during the game, where I'd get the ball from a lineout and pass to Timmy Horan, then he'd start to go across field with his centre partner, Jason Little, almost toward the corner flag. Then Campo would come from the open side and cut back late and counter-intuitively go inside, beating the defence, we hoped. I decided to call the 'S' move. There were two reasons for doing that. One, we'd been successful with it throughout the game. Two, if Campo got caught, at least he'd be near the forwards instead of being wide out on his own. I wanted to make absolutely sure we secured the ball. Without it, the game was over.

TIM HORAN: Michael was a much better running flyhalf than he was given credit for and he had amazing awareness. He was quicker than you thought too, but—more importantly—he knew exactly when to run, where to run and when to pass. As his inside centre, you didn't even have to worry about his pass. You just ran for the gap and you just knew that the ball would be there.

So we ran 'S' and Campo came back in as he was supposed to, but he didn't get very far before getting caught. He was normally like most backs: he would get caught in amongst the forwards and then would get himself out of there. But if you watch a replay, Campo actually stayed in there. He was pulling towards the Irish goal line—'Come on, push!' with Simon Poidevin latched onto him.

It seemed to be an important barometer. I thought, 'Shit, if *he* was listening, *everybody* was.' We got the put-in to the scrum on the left-hand side of the field and Timmy came up to me and said, 'Drop goal?' I immediately said 'No.' A drop goal would have given us a draw, and what I didn't know at the time was that a draw would have got us through on a try count. I thought the match would go into extra time. I said, 'We're going to do *this*', and Timmy didn't even question me. I had a very clear plan in my head. We just had to execute it. Timmy just said 'Okay' and trotted back. He believed in me. They *all* believed in me.

BOB DWYER: Michael's leadership skills rocketed to the forefront. For me it's his true single moment of absolute greatness. He took control of the situation and led the other fourteen guys: 'You do this; you do that. Finished.' And he did it. From the leadership angle, and we'll never be overplaying it, it was the defining moment in his career. It was made even more amazing by the fact that, because he's modest and self-effacing, he's not really a natural leader. He gets cross, but it's how that anger comes across that defines leadership. I don't know how to say this nicely, but sometimes he just has the shits and that doesn't always come across positively. But on this occasion he led the team out of defeat. I can't speak more highly of it. I thought about it afterwards and said to myself, 'If he had gone on to the field as captain, would the result have been the same?' Or was it the demands of the situation at that moment that excluded negative thoughts from his mind at that time? When he was put in a crisis, his leadership came out.

All week we'd been looking at the Irish midfield to see exactly how they defended, what the patterns were. We came up with a move to take advantage of that and it had worked all the way through the game. 'Working' hadn't always turned into tries, of course, but we'd always made ground and made breaks. There was always some kind of progress. In my mind, it didn't matter what stage of the game it was. It would have been easy to panic and reach for something ambitious that we hadn't rehearsed. But this was the move we'd practised and this was what we were going to do.

The scrum was good. Solid. We got the ball and off we went.

The move worked well until Brendan Mullin tackled Jason from behind. The move involved Timmy missing Jason to pass to Marty Roebuck, and then Jason would loop around Marty into the open. That was the theory.

But Brendan Mullin must have worked the move out. He saw it coming. He defended in the way we expected at the outset, but then he somehow managed to follow Jason and run him down from behind, almost before he got the ball. Instead of making ground Jason just managed to unload to Campo, who by that time had a little bit of space. Nine times out of ten in situations like that, he scores. But somehow the Irish managed to pull him down. My role was to just be there, supporting, and I *was* there, just like I had been throughout that game and in most other games. Then, when Campo threw one of his better passes—in other words he rolled it along the ground—I picked it up and dived over in the tackle. We'd made it.

I heard the whistle go and all our guys were yelling and screaming. And then there was deathly silence. I thought, 'Something's wrong. What's happened?' Then I realised what had happened. We had destroyed the hopes of a nation.

Then I had to walk back and take the kick at goal. It didn't matter; we were going to win the game. I was physically and mentally exhausted. Jim Fleming came over and said, 'Can you hurry up?' I said, 'Mate, I can hardly lift my legs, let alone kick.'

My enduring memory of the dressing room afterwards is how incredibly ecstatic Nick and Bob Dwyer were. I'd never seen them so emotional. Up in the stands, they must have been thinking, 'We're out. We're going home,' and the worst part of it was that there was absolutely nothing they could do about it.

BOB DWYER: When Michael came off he was absolutely bubbling. He was like a six-year-old kid on Christmas morning. He was so excited that he was shaking and the words were pouring out of his mouth. It was fantastic and I'd never seen him like that coming off the footie field.

I was obviously elated, but I was also pragmatic. I just thought, 'That's what needed to be done'—and the team responded magnificently. There was never a question asked—they just did the job. That's the sign of a great team. Whenever I stand up and talk in a business setting, and I don't do it too often, I sometimes refer to Dublin as a blueprint of how to approach an extremely testing situation—in life, as well as rugby. You prepare as best you can and then, when it matters, under pressure, that preparation pays off when your team delivers. It's a wonderful example of achieving a pre-determined goal.

I'm incredibly proud of those four minutes, not just because we won the game and eventually won the tournament. What excites me more about it is that I was able to come up with a plan and clearly transmit that information to the team—'If we win, we win. If we don't, we don't. But this is the move we've practised. Let's execute it.' And we did.

As a player, that was the pinnacle passage of play of my entire career right there. I'm in charge and then, in the midst of all that pressure and mayhem, with an entire nation against us, I'm able to come up with a clear plan, articulate it then produce it—it just doesn't get any better.

The fact that I scored the winning try was irrelevant; it just happened to be me. It could have been anybody; I'd still feel the same pride about what I did that day. The game for me was all about the decisions, the planning and the final execution. This'll sound strange, maybe, but as a single moment, it eclipsed beating England in the final. Even now, the whole of Ireland remembers it. I still get messages on Twitter about it, people saying, 'Damn you, Michael Lynagh! I'll never forget that try', accompanied by an image of me going over in the corner. It's always good-natured stuff; that's how the Irish are. It's just that most Irish people who saw the game remember exactly where they were when I scored the try. And Gordon Hamilton and I are forever linked. It became for many Irish the Gordon Hamilton/Michael Lynagh game.

YOU'D THINK THAT PICKING myself up for a game against New Zealand in the semis would have been difficult after that. Honestly, it wasn't at all. If anything, the resolve we'd drawn from pulling the Ireland win out in the dying seconds only reinforced my feeling that we needed to go on and make it really mean something by winning the World Cup. I'm not saying that not winning the World Cup would have rendered Dublin meaningless, not at all. But I knew that chances to win the World Cup don't come along very often so you've got to grab them when they do.

BOB DWYER: It's hard to say whether the Ireland game was what won us the World Cup, but what I can say with absolute certainty is that, if we hadn't beaten Ireland, we definitely wouldn't have done it! A lot of good judges said, 'The Wallabies are now favourites. Any team that can get themselves out of a situation in the manner in which they did has got all the answers.' The Irish press definitely followed that line.

So we were motivated for it. It wasn't a difficult situation to assess either. Both teams knew that whoever won it would be favourites to win the World Cup. The All Blacks, as they normally are, were pretty confident. They were almost dismissive in a 'Well, we're the best team, get out of our way' type of way. It was a great attitude to have. It's an aura and they bank on that. Whether that ever translated into complacency, I don't know. It could also be that the '91 All Black team was simply at the end of a great cycle for them. That happens to all winning teams.

Before we played them, though, we all needed time to recharge the batteries a bit and Ireland's an ideal spot to do it. Some guys went on tours around Dublin; Nick and I and a few of the others went for some golf at Portmarnock, on the coast. It really is a beautiful part of the world and the Irish people were now on our side. Instead of siding with the All Blacks, they almost seemed to take a 'Well, we almost beat you so we're now on your side' stance when it came to the semi-final. That made a massive difference. Also, unlike the All Blacks, who made themselves pretty unapproachable to the public during that week, we were the opposite. We'd be out walking in Dublin, talking to the fans and signing autographs. It all helped sway the locals in our favour.

As it happened, the first half against New Zealand in the semi was maybe the best half of rugby I was ever part of for Australia. As someone who was in that '86 Bledisloe Cup team, that's really saying something. We just blew them away. Campo, in particular, was absolutely terrific. Then, in the second half, when they threw the kitchen sink at us, as we fully expected them to, it was just a matter of holding on. All hands on deck.

There was a moment in the second half when their big second-rower Gary Whetton made a break down the right-hand side. As usual, I was coming across in cover. It was me and him. If I missed the tackle, he scored. Gary was a big guy and very quick for his size and had about thirty metres of build-up on me. I just remember grabbing him around one leg, holding on and dragging him into touch. I thought to myself, 'There you go—that wasn't a bad tackle.'

ALL I REMEMBER ABOUT the build-up to the final at Twickenham was that I was terribly nervous. As usual, I wasn't remotely concerned about the playing aspect—the decision-making, the collisions or the tactics. It was the goal-kicking that was making me feel physically sick.

I went down to Twickenham the day before the final to do some kicking practice. Alone. As I walked back to my mark each time, I looked at the posts at each corner of the ground at pitch level. One would be pointing this way, and the one on the other side would be pointing that way. You'd feel the wind in front of you, but when you looked at these posts, they were going in different directions.

In those days Twickenham wasn't completely enclosed. There were gaps at the corners. So when you kicked, it felt like the wind was going one way, but actually it was doing the exact opposite. I worked out that the wind would enter the stadium at a corner and then bounce off the stands and come back at you. It took ages to figure it out, and the way I finally did it was by looking right up on top of the stand at where the flags were flying. They were all going the same way. That was the true direction of the wind and you had to trust that completely, regardless of what it felt like.

GRANT FOX: One of the hardest disciplines in goal-kicking is to trust what you actually know, even if it's exactly the opposite of what you feel. I've stood in front of countless kicks at Eden Park where it feels like the wind is coming from the left. The logical response to that would be to aim a little left to compensate. But I knew that the wind was actually from the right and really I had to be aiming right. There's such a conflict there. But you have to trust what you actually know.

Even though I felt I'd learned a few things about Twickenham, I was terribly nervous that night. It had become a habit for me to lie in bed the night before big games, mentally rehearsing my kicks. I used it as a means of falling asleep. I'd gone from the fifteen-metre line on one side, to the fifteen-metre line on the other side when I was practising. Then I'd done the same at the other end. To the point that, by the time I was rehearsing it in my mind, I knew exactly what the signage was, the colour of the dot in the middle of the sign, the colour of the flags and where they were blowing. It was very detailed in my mind. I'd compare it to counting sheep as a way to fall asleep. It relaxed me and stopped me worrying about wider issues like: 'How's it going to go tomorrow?'

The team was based at a hotel out in Weybridge called Oatlands Park. I liked getting up and going for a walk in the morning before most big games. Sometimes I'd try to have a bit of a kick. I found an area of ground near the hotel so I went there alone the morning of the final for a bit with a ball. There were no posts or anything, just this open piece of ground. Every time I kicked the ball, I'd have to go and chase after it. I felt a little silly. Then I noticed this nearby hill that sloped down to a creek. It wasn't far away. I thought, 'That's the idea. I'll go down to the bottom, kick it up and it'll just roll back down the hill to me.' So that's what I did.

On the bus on the way to the ground I went through the whole series of mental rehearsals again. It was my way of dealing with the nerves. The result was that when I actually got there in the match situation, I'd kicked that goal already. I'd physically done it the day before and I'd done it ten times mentally. I'd *been* there. There could be no surprises.

So when I was awarded a kick in the match—one that was way out on the touchline—I didn't panic. I just thought, 'This is fine. I've kicked it already.' I had, and I slotted it in at a very important stage of the game. I kicked the majority of my goals that day because of what I'd learned about the wind the day before. If I hadn't practised, I probably would have missed them all. On that occasion I executed when it mattered and we went on to win the World Cup.

Interestingly, I've never actually watched that entire 1991 final. I've seen highlights, but never the whole game. My father was over staying with us in April of 2015 and I thought that it might be really nice for all of us—three generations of Lynaghs—to sit and watch a recording that I'd made earlier from an ESPN rerun. What surprised me was that, early in the game, we were awarded a penalty. It wasn't far out and it was reasonably straight. As the kids were watching with me they said, 'Oh Dad, you'd better get this one …' I didn't even come close to getting it. I didn't just miss it; I missed it by miles. The commentator said something like, 'Even Lynagh must be feeling the pressure.' I have no recollection of the kick at all. All I remember are the harder ones I kicked at important moments in the game.

EIGHT

GIULIANO'S DAUGHTER

I'D HAD SEVERAL APPROACHES from Italian clubs over the years and I'd always politely declined—just said, 'No thanks.'

The timing had never felt right, usually for the same two reasons. First, I wanted to play for Queensland and Australia and had no desire to jeopardise that in any way by being detached from that scene. Secondly, in managing the Queensland office of the New Zealand-based property investment group Robert Jones Investments, I had a job that I was happy with and didn't want to jeopardise that either. I thought, 'Life's good—no need to change things too much.'

The thing that changed my mind back in 1991—when I was approached by the guys from Benetton Treviso—was that I'd realised that, while I'd enjoyed every aspect of my life, I couldn't ignore the fact that I'd been doing the same things, running around the same paddocks, playing for the same teams, for ten years. There was nothing negative about arriving at that conclusion; it was just one of those moments when you know that you're standing at a fork in the road—one that says, in bold letters: 'Maybe there's more to life?'

With hindsight, knowing that going to Italy completely changed my world, I'm glad I was smart enough to recognise what I was being presented with at the time. Even as a young man I always tried to take a breath and allow these realisations to sink in. Then, when I'd done that and weighed up the various options available to me, I made a decision and lived with it.

With that in mind, I decided that 1991 was a logical point in my career to take six months out to do something completely different. It seemed right to break the cycle. In those days, with professional rugby still a few years down the line, the inducement to play overseas was not financial, but simply the challenge of playing rugby and living in another country.

Fortunately, that inducement was worth something to me. I like travelling and experiencing new cultures, and touring with Australia had taught me a lot about that. But in a tour party you're in a controlled environment. And it's a good one: you're representing your country with a great bunch of rugby players who are also your friends—each of you with a whole raft of common values to uphold. The green and gold meant something when we travelled in a group. But playing club rugby abroad meant something different. This time it was about me, and my opportunities to explore the world. Hopefully, Australia would still be there whenever I went back and would welcome me. Saying that, the decision to go to Italy was still not an easy one to make.

But it all aligned in April of 1991. While I was playing in the Hong Kong Sevens, Fabrizio Gaetaniello, the director of rugby at Treviso, and Amerino Zatta, a senior figure in Benetton, flew out to meet me and it was then that I decided to make the move—to commit to this new challenge. I suppose I'd already decided that after the World Cup in October could be the right time to go and spend six months in Italy. Obviously I didn't know then that we'd go on and *win* the World Cup, but my decision honestly wouldn't have changed either way. If anything, winning only reinforced my sense that one part of my life was drawing to a close and another exciting phase was about to begin.

A conversation with my boss, Robert Jones, confirmed that I was making the right decision, because when I went in to his office to discuss the plan he said: 'If you don't go, I'm going!' Then he added: 'And by the way, when you come back I'd like you to work with me in Sydney.' So I actually got promoted at the same time as telling him I was leaving for a while. Not every day is as good as that one!

Instead of being a complete step into the unknown, it initially seemed as if there was a comforting degree of familiarity about moving to Italy. I'd been to Treviso while on tour with Queensland in 1986 and thought I knew exactly what I was getting into. By any standards it was a picture-postcard town and the facilities from a rugby perspective were outstanding: a state-of-the-art gym, restaurant and golf driving range, for starters. So just two weeks after we'd won a World Cup at Twickenham for Australia, there I was, playing in my first game for Treviso at L'Aquila, an eight-hour bus journey away and the venue at which I'd made my Wallaby debut in 1983 against the Italy A side.

L'Aquila, historically, was an extremely tough place to play. The guys were big, physical. We were one of the best teams in

Italy, but even we were a little nervous about the game. The instructions I received from the coach, the legendary Pierre Villepreux, on the bus before my first appearance were basic, to say the least. 'Yes' and 'no', I knew. Then he taught me 'left' and 'right' so that I could at least let my halfback know which way to go. Then he said, 'If you want to try to motivate the forwards a little bit, just say *"Spingi!"*' That simply meant 'Push!'—it was hardly technical stuff. That was the extent of my Italian when I played my first match. My vocabulary definitely had scope for improvement.

I'll never forget sitting in the dressing room beforehand, as we tried to motivate ourselves. I felt like a fish out of water. I was listening to what was going on without really understanding much of it. One of the guys was prowling around the dressing room, shaking his fist and shouting: *'Dai ragazzi! Dai ragazzi!'*

'Die?' I thought to myself. 'That seems a bit over the top, doesn't it?'

I was all for giving it a go but I wasn't prepared to stake my life on a game! I remember asking one of the guys what it meant and he laughed and told me that our enthusiastic teammate was saying 'Come on' or 'Let's go!'

Despite my basic familiarity with the surroundings, to call my initial weeks in Italy a smooth transition wouldn't really be accurate. In day-to-day, practical terms it was anything but. The language barrier was a bigger obstacle than I'd imagined, and with new faces all around me it felt more like I'd dropped in from another planet. It was exactly the type of situation that I don't generally take kindly to. The awkwardness was reinforced by the fact that I couldn't even pronounce my halfback partner's name, far less hold a conversation with him! I was certainly outside my comfort zone and in some ways that was no bad thing. After all, I was twenty-eight years old—a World Cup winner with a decade of relative predictability under my belt. I thought to myself, 'You wanted a challenge, mate. You've got one.'

My habitual response to that kind of unease is to do my best to solve the problem. So at a very early stage I asked Benetton if I could have Italian lessons. It was my first step towards self-sufficiency. They agreed. I willingly went to the classes every day and at training at night the guys would ask: 'So, what did you learn today?' Normally they spoke to each other in dialect, but with me they made a point of speaking correct Italian. That really helped me. I appreciated it and I think, from their perspective, they appreciated that I was willing to try to integrate more.

As I was a foreigner in a new country, people often came up to me after games to say hello, trying to be welcoming and friendly. After one of the first matches I played in, an elegant gentleman approached me. He spoke pretty good English and he said, 'Nice to meet you, Michael. I'm Giuliano and I love rugby.' He was very pleasant and seemed to have a good knowledge of the game. He added, 'And by the way, my daughter did an exchange in Florida and speaks very good English. You'll have to come over for dinner one night.'

Initially, I didn't think too much of it. By nature, most Italians are very open and generous, so friendliness of this kind wasn't exactly unusual. I thanked him and then, two weeks later, the same thing happened again, except this time Giuliano finished the conversation slightly differently, adding: 'And by the way, my daughter said to say hello.'

Unbeknownst to me, Giuliano and his daughter (whose name, I had learned, was Isabella) had watched me play against Ireland in the World Cup. They'd definitely picked the right game! Apparently they'd been very excited, and Giuliano had said, 'See that guy who just scored that try? Well, he's the one coming to Treviso to play this season.'

'He looks nice. He probably doesn't speak much Italian,' Isabella apparently said, 'Let's have him over for dinner sometime.'

ISABELLA LYNAGH: I saw Michael on TV while watching with my father. I had always been a rugby fan because of my father's interest in the club. I saw him score the try and when my father told me Michael was coming to play at Treviso, I said out loud, 'Ah, he does look good! I wouldn't mind meeting him.' I was going out with someone else at the time, though, and my reason for wanting to meet Michael was to learn better English. Of course, Michael never actually came over for dinner and the reason was that I had a boyfriend.

These post-match chats went on for a good many weeks. Giuliano would say similar things each time we talked and over time I got to know him and his wife, Daniela, pretty well, although I never went over to their place for dinner. Isabella never came to the games, or if she did I didn't meet her. Actually, when I think about it, this went on for almost the whole season!

Inevitably, as time passed, I started to develop a mental portrait of this seemingly mythical girl in my mind.

'What sort of girl sends her father to say hello, but never actually comes to meet me?' I wondered.

It didn't really make sense. I had a vision, in the absence of anything tangible, of a traditional-looking Italian girl: black hair, maybe quite big, shrouded in old-fashioned black clothing. I really hoped I was wrong.

Just before the club semi-finals, I went for lunch with some friends to a beautiful village called Asolo, in the foothills of the Dolomites. We had a very nice meal, and afterwards, as Italians do, we went for a walk through the stunning town centre, which was closed to traffic. As we were strolling among the crowds, I noticed a girl in the group that was coming towards us. I thought, 'She looks nice.' Gianni Zanon—the fellow I was walking with—nodded to her and said hello as we passed.

I said, 'Who was that?'

I turned and watched her walk away.

Gianni said, 'Oh, that's a friend of the committee's daughter.'

I gathered that meant she was one of the club member's daughters. It didn't register to me at the time, but that was Isabella. Also unbeknownst to me, she—at that same moment—had commented to one of her friends: 'Oh, that's the Australian rugby player—he's nice.' We reported these stories later, but at the time we didn't know each other and passed by as strangers.

A few weeks later we played in the finals against Naas Botha's Rovigo side in Padova. We won, I scored two tries and it was a fantastic game of rugby all round. We ran the ball from almost everywhere. We blitzed them. It couldn't have been scripted any better. When we emerged from the dressing room we got a typical Italian victory greeting from the fans: hordes of people were chanting and waving flags. Afterwards, as we made our way through the car park of celebrating fans towards where the bus was waiting, I ran into Giuliano and his wife, Daniela. They were hugging me, congratulating me on the win, when they suddenly stopped and said, 'By the way, Isabella is here today ...'

I thought, 'Oh, that's all I need right now.' I was picturing that old-fashioned, slightly dowdy Italian girl I'd imagined.

'... and here she is!' Giuliano announced, revealing a beautiful long-haired blonde girl who spoke perfect English.

I thought: 'Oh my God!' I actually said: 'Why didn't you tell me?!'

'I've been trying for the last six months!' Giuliano replied.

ISABELLA LYNAGH: I ended up at the final with friends, one of whom was my boyfriend. We had a falling out and, instead of meeting me at the stadium exit as agreed, he left without me. I was stuck with my parents, being sulky, and that's when I met Michael. It was pure fate. As soon as we met, it was like a lightning bolt passed through me. I knew he was trouble.

Isabella didn't really know what to say to me, but she eventually asked me if I wouldn't mind signing her ticket. I remember signing it 'Con amicizia [with friendship] from Michael Lynagh' and she still carries it with her today. We chatted for the few moments before the team was due to leave for a celebratory dinner at a beautiful restaurant outside Treviso. Friends and supporters were planning to congregate there also, and so I asked Isabella if she'd like to join us. I thought, 'What have I got to lose?' As it turned out, her parents had planned to go there already, so she came with them and we spent the evening chatting, just the two of us.

Something I didn't know at the time was that Isabella was at the rugby that day with her parents because she'd had a fight with her boyfriend—a boyfriend I had no knowledge of whatsoever, I should probably add. Apparently he didn't like rugby, so on the few occasions that they'd come along to games, they'd left directly afterwards. Now it all made sense and it seemed that perhaps fate had intervened on my behalf.

'Lovely to meet you,' I said as she was leaving. 'By the way, a friend of mine is having a going-away barbecue for me tomorrow; why don't you come along?'

'I think my parents are coming to that so maybe I'll come with them,' she answered.

I thought, 'So far so good.'

Isabella did appear the next day and, again, we chatted pleasantly all afternoon until, at around four o clock, I had to leave to catch a flight back to Brisbane. We were starting the build-up to a Test match against a touring Scotland side in Sydney on June 13th 1992. As far as I was concerned, my time in Italy was over. After all, I had a new job waiting for me and I'd be playing rugby for my country again in little more than a week. In my mind, life was about to return to normal.

ISABELLA LYNAGH: I went to the barbecue and we talked for about seven hours. It was like we knew each other already. I used to play competitive tennis and to talk to an elite sportsman at the peak of his career, who had just won the World Cup, was a big attraction for me. I found the psychological aspect very interesting.

I REMEMBER THERE BEING a little bit of talk about me and Campo—who was also playing rugby in Italy—coming back to

Australia and walking straight into the Test team. Bob Dwyer picked us for the Scotland game and I remember John Connolly, my coach at Queensland, being reasonably critical of that. It wasn't a big thing, but I do remember being a bit discomforted. In reality, John was probably just stirring the pot to unsettle Bob Dwyer a little, nothing much more than that.

I was sensitive to the feelings of the guys who'd been playing hard all season at home. I certainly had no intention of upsetting anyone or doing anything other than playing fair, particularly as I'd gone to Italy with the blessing of both Queensland and the Australian Rugby Union. In those pre-contract days, nobody could have stopped me going anyway, and we all knew that. Equally, I knew from the start that the potential penalty for playing abroad was that I wouldn't get picked. I wouldn't be under the selectors' noses. I just hoped that the way I handled myself in combination with coming back in good form would be enough to secure my place, and that generally proved to be the case throughout my career in Italy. It didn't help that quite a few influential people back home didn't consider playing Italian rugby to be valid preparation. Granted, the standard of rugby in the lower Italian leagues probably wasn't up to much. But I was playing in the top tier, *winning* in the top tier—it was more than competitive.

Incidentally, I always got on very well with John Connolly and he was a very, very good forwards coach. We never had any run-ins other than when he dropped me as captain in 1989, and even that was okay. I usually saw people's reasons for making decisions, even when they negatively impacted me.

John was very forwards-orientated, and was good at getting them drilled. But when it came to the backs he used to defer to

John Brass, the backs coach. I remember one particular team meeting when Connolly said, 'We're going to win the ball, the forwards will drive', all that kind of thing. 'Then you just give the ball to Michael and he'll do what he does.' It was pretty simplistic, but I took it as a compliment.

He used to have a laugh about me being late for training at Ballymore too. My office was in the city and while it wasn't far to Ballymore as the crow flies, at the time I was trying to get there, I usually got caught in traffic. All the other guys, like Timmy Horan, would be there at 5.30pm for a bit of a kick, a pass or a team meeting. But training didn't officially start until 6pm.

Seemingly there was a standing joke at my expense.

John would pull all the guys onto the pitch at 6pm, and nine times out of ten I wasn't quite there. Then, when he saw my car appear over the hill, he'd look at his watch and say, 'Okay guys, it's Noddy time!'

GIVEN THE HIGH COST of international phone calls in those days before emails and text messages, letters and faxes were the only ways Isabella and I could keep in contact while I was back in Australia. It's funny; my sons nowadays say things like, 'What's a fax machine?' At that time I considered myself very lucky to have one at home. But the only one Isabella had access to was the one at her father's office, so I'd ring her very quickly, barely long enough to get out the words: 'I'm sending a fax … *now.*' That way she could rush down to the office and intercept it before anyone else got to it.

In this way, in the odd spare minutes between my new job and rugby commitments, we continued to get to know each other. Eventually, after a few months, Treviso asked if I'd like to return for another season. I had every intention of going back to Italy; there was no doubt in my mind. But I was in a slightly awkward position with my boss and my first thought was that I needed to be one hundred per cent upfront and honest with him. I loved the job, but I wanted to go to Italy for six months even more.

ISABELLA LYNAGH: The club knew that I was in touch with Michael so eventually they came to me and said, 'Do you think he'd be interested in coming back?' I said, 'Well, you better talk to him. But I hope so!'

It was also in the back of my mind that Australia had a three-week tour to South Africa in August and then, later in the year, another lengthy trip to Ireland and Wales. All of this combined would represent a lot of time away from the office, and in the case of the Wallaby tours I would be *paid* by Robert Jones to be away from the office. That made me uneasy.

As much as I loved my new role at Robert Jones Investments and the generous amount of flexibility my boss gave me, rather than stringing him along, I decided that it was probably the right time to part ways on good terms. It was a decision I've always felt was the right one. Better to do as you would be done by, I always think.

NINE

A NEW ROLE

I ALWAYS CONSIDERED SOUTH Africa to be a very intense place from a rugby point of view. My father took me to one of the more controversial Test matches in rugby history, between the Springboks and the Wallabies in Brisbane in 1971. I was only seven at the time and remember nothing of the game whatsoever, but I do remember sensing the danger in the air. I was right to feel that way. A state of emergency had been declared in Queensland in an attempt to quell the anti-apartheid demonstrations that overshadowed the whole Springbok tour.

Fast-forward twenty-odd years to the summer of 1992 and I was part of the first Australian touring party to set foot in South Africa since the late 1960s. It was a big occasion, not least because the All Blacks were there at the same time.

Unlike in Australia, where rugby union is not the number one winter sport, the game is very much part of daily life in South Africa. Back in 1992 the white population lived and breathed it. Then they lived it a bit more. That's no different from how it used to be in Wales and still is in New Zealand, but because the Springboks had been exiled from the world stage for so long, the excitement and intensity we encountered there were on another level from anything we'd previously experienced. To add spice to the mix, we were arriving there as reigning World Champions, and in the eyes of the bullish locals that meant we were there to be scrutinised and there to be beaten.

All we'd heard about back in Australia was how volatile things were in South Africa. While the political climate was certainly more promising than it had been for many years, it wasn't as if there had been an overnight transformation from the dark days of apartheid to the kind of inclusive society we were accustomed to. With security with us wherever we went, South Africa—by any normal standards—was an intimidating and strangely exciting environment to be in and we definitely had to tread lightly at times.

I remember one incident early in the tour, in Pretoria. We were at a function, drinking wine and chatting. Nick Farr-Jones and I were making polite small talk with some local bigwig when I asked, for no reason other than to fill a void in the conversation, 'So, how many people are there in South Africa?'

This guy said, 'Well, if you count the blacks, there's forty million. If you don't count them, there are just five million.'

He wasn't smiling.

Nick and I looked at each other quizzically. We couldn't believe what we were hearing.

Nick said, 'Well, why wouldn't you count them?'

The guy just stared at him blankly.

We never did get the answer.

Then, during a free afternoon, we were enjoying a barbecue arranged for the squad in a game park. It was a beautiful day, a relaxed atmosphere. We were having a beer or two when some local fans came over to chat, bringing items for us to sign. One of them went up to Willie Ofahengaue and said, 'Hey boy! Sign this would you, boy?'

The charitable view would be that it was probably no different from me saying something like, 'Hey mate, would you sign this?' But the turn of phrase didn't come across well in the context. It sounded really bad. We all sat there for a moment, not sure what might happen next.

Now, if you don't already know, Willie O is of Tongan descent, seventeen stone plus and six foot three. A really big unit. Willie never said very much. You had to really push him. But when spoken to like that, he isn't going to be happy. He looked up, and for a fleeting moment it looked like there might be a major incident, but in the end, to his eternal credit, he just quietly said, 'Please do not call me that again. My name is Willie.'

As strange as it might sound, I don't think there was any real animosity or nastiness behind either of these two incidents. It was more of an ingrained cultural thing that needed to be addressed through education, though in the second instance the turn of phrase needed to change and change fast. But I guess if you told me to stop saying the word 'mate' it would probably take me a little while because I'm so used to saying it. I'll give the guy the benefit of the doubt; maybe it was so habitual with him that it would take time before his mouth and brain caught up with the new South Africa.

NICK FARR-JONES: South Africa in 1992 was still a very divided country. I got woken at 1am the morning after South Africa played New Zealand and was told that the ANC [African National Congress] were having a meeting to discuss withdrawing their support for our tour. They'd asked for three conditions to be observed prior to all tour matches. First, the non-waving of the old flag. Secondly, the non-playing of the old anthem and, finally, the observance of a minute's silence for victims of township violence. When we were at the All Black match in Johannesburg, all these conditions were unbelievably breached. So the morning after that match we woke the team and said, 'Guys, we're still going to training but pack your bags.' It came very close to our tour being abandoned, but the then sports minister in South Africa stepped in and said, in reference to the three conditions: 'Give them one more chance.' Our tour was that close to ending and there were two planes ready to fly us out of the country if need be.

The first game of the tour was against Western Transvaal in Potchefstroom—very much a rural Afrikaner stronghold. The locals were, shall we say, fervent. When the bus was being driven through the car park at Olën Park, the supporters were shouting and hammering on its sides—there were really intense scenes. I thought, 'So this is what a boxer feels like, walking through the crowd to the ring.'

I remember that Nick stood up at the front of the bus—he had a serious look on his face. 'Look guys, this is very different for us. Concentrate on the job and don't get intimidated by the atmosphere.'

He was right—we knew what the job at hand was. But you couldn't help being unsettled. We'd heard about how huge the South African players were, how good they were. That aside, we had no idea whatsoever about their style of play—it was all an unknown quantity for us. As it turned out, we won the game fairly comfortably, but it was very tough, very physical and extremely intimidating.

After we won the game, the head-games began. The words 'What a great side Australia is. No wonder they beat us—they're the reigning World Champions' were never heard. Instead it was, 'Yeah, well you're not really World Champions unless you beat Northern Transvaal.'

We beat Northern Transvaal.

And then it was the same thing with the Eastern Province, and so on. Even when we'd won all of our three provincial games, two of them by pretty wide margins it should be said, the doubters still wouldn't lie down.

'*Not* until you've beaten South Africa.'

BOB DWYER: There were actual posters all over Cape Town that said, 'You're not the World Champions until you beat us.'

A score of 26–3 later, after the Newlands Test match, everyone was a little bit quieter. We outmatched the Springboks in every discipline—particularly upfront. But at no point were any of these games easy, even if the scoreboards suggested they might have been. These were sides with a lot of strengths and even more to prove, but there were definitely aspects of their game that reflected their lengthy spell in isolation. We needed to show them we meant business. I'll never forget a tackle Willie O made on the Springbok hooker Uli Schmidt early in the Test. Schmidt was a big guy with a low centre of gravity. He could run a bit too, when he'd worked up a head of steam. Willie dropped his shoulder and buried him—stopped him dead in his tracks, right in front of me. It was the kind of moment that makes you breathe a sigh of relief and think, 'I reckon we're going to be all right here.' Just as well Willie tackled him—I was next in line if he'd missed. Willie was a silent presence on the field but he worked extremely hard. When we were calling moves, we'd tell him what it was and he'd just nod. He didn't discuss it; he just went and did what was required every single time. He never, ever, missed an assignment.

With hindsight, South Africa were a little predictable defensively—you could read them. You could probably explain that when you consider that the players had been defending exclusively against one another on a weekly basis for years. It was as if Queensland played New South Wales or Leicester played Bath every weekend. Eventually it reaches a point where you're only as good as your opposition—'Oh, not *this* move again—we've seen all that before.'

And if that opposition doesn't have any outside influence either, predictable patterns—and responses to those patterns—develop almost subconsciously. You know the players you're playing against inside out—what they're good at and what they're not so good at—and that's what seemed to have been happening in South African domestic rugby. It was unavoidable. They were in a goldfish bowl. When a touring side like Australia turned up—battle hardened, *Test match* hardened—they were presented with a whole new set of problems: pace, style, defensive strategy and so on. It caught them by surprise, and understandably so.

On reflection, the boot could easily have been on the other foot. We'd only seen occasional footage of Currie Cup games, so it's possible that they could have caught us out. Their domestic game could have been miles ahead of what we were doing and we could have been whitewashed 4–0. Instead of us saying, 'Yeah, we beat you too', it would have been, 'Oh my God, these guys were sleeping giants all along.' As it stood, though—after being beaten by New Zealand and us on successive weekends—it was clear that the South Africans had hoped they were at a certain level in 1992, but that they weren't quite there. Not yet. We'd learn of their progress the following summer when they came to Australia.

HAVING HANDED IN MY notice with Robert Jones Investments, I decided to return to Italy following the Wallaby tour to Wales and Ireland in the northern autumn of 1992, my first tour as captain of my country. I was the logical choice; there really wasn't anyone else. How did I feel about the new role? Well, I knew for sure that the outgoing skipper, Nick Farr-Jones, and I were very different personalities. Nick was always more extroverted and vocal. That was his style and I admired it. I'd think, 'Good on you.'

NICK FARR-JONES: I always got on well with [the Wallaby coach] Bob Dwyer. We debated and argued a lot but we always ended up back on the same page. I never really felt that Michael was totally comfortable with Bob. Bob came from the Randwick, running-rugby, ball-in-hand background, and I always thought he perceived Michael to be central to the typical Queensland ethos, which was very positional—with a fair bit of kicking deployed to get out of your own half.

But I always felt that I was as much a leader on the field as Nick was—albeit with a completely different approach. Over many years of playing together we had been an effective halves pairing who knew each other's game inside out, we also complemented each other well as people, in that we both brought slightly different qualities to the table.

BOB DYWER: Our relationship was quite mature with a strong degree of trust. Certainly on my part there was confidence in Michael as a captain. I felt we could talk to each other about any subject. Nick was a bit more forthright than Michael was, however. He'd come to me and say things like, 'You think I can play better, don't you?' I'd reply, 'Seeing as you ask, yes, I do think you can play better.' Michael would never come to me and say something like that.

One thing I knew I needed to do when I became captain was speak up a little. While being overly vocal isn't my style, I knew that the team as a whole needed me to come out of my shell a bit more. I was nervous about doing that and to help with the transition I relied on the hooker and vice-captain, Phil Kearns, in a way that perfectly complemented my strengths. Kearnsy was a typical front-row forward: gregarious and a good motivator of people on the field. While I made a big effort to engage more with the team than I previously had under Nick's captaincy, I knew where my strengths lay and where other people were perhaps better placed to deploy theirs. I relied on other people too. David Wilson was another forward to whom I delegated some of the team management roles. In the backs I included guys like Timmy Horan and Jason Little as well as David Campese. That was always the best way of managing Campo: make him feel that he was involved in team decision-making.

I was more comfortable in a role where I was the less obvious voice of authority. I was the captain of the team and nobody was in any doubt about that—I'd proved in Dublin in 1991 that I had all the attributes needed. But on occasions I preferred to delegate some of the man-management roles to my vice-captain. Kearnsy and I turned out to be a good combination and the tour went well until I dislocated my shoulder making a cover tackle against Ireland at Lansdowne Road, somewhat ironically. From a playing perspective the tour was over for me.

With a season in Italy around the corner and with the injury unlikely to properly repair simply with rest and time (that anyway I just didn't have), I returned to Brisbane and underwent an operation to repair the injury before rejoining the tour in Wales as non-playing captain. The shoulder was delicate; still pretty painful. And the medical people always sow a seed of doubt: 'Take it easy; don't rush it. There's a lot going on in there.'

I RETURNED TO ITALY in December of 1992, thinking, 'This is going to be an interesting few months.' When I weighed it all up, the main reason for going back to Treviso was remarkably simple: I'd loved the whole experience—it was a no-brainer to go back. Yes, for language reasons the first three months had been difficult, but once the fog lifted, as it had felt to me, I really enjoyed everything. I felt at home there. Not just that, looking at things from a purely rugby perspective, the year had been a success. I'd personally played well and we'd won the final. All was good. I could order dinner in a restaurant or a beer in a bar, and while I wouldn't say I was fluent or even proficient in the language at that time, I certainly knew enough to converse and get by on a day-to-day basis.

Prior to coming to Italy, I'd never been a great food connoisseur. I was very much from the 'If I'm hungry, I'll eat something' school of thinking. I'd always been of the view that food was just food. But you can't survive like that for very long in a country where food, wine and the enjoyment of sharing them are part and parcel of the daily culture. As time went on, I started to appreciate that things like food and wine were pretty important.

I remember telling the guys at training one night, 'I went to this restaurant last night.' They said, 'Oh really, what did you have?' I said, 'Pasta and then some meat.' They laughed and said, 'No, but what did you really have? *What* was the pasta? What *kind* of a sauce was it? How was it cooked?' I'd never really considered those details before, but I was gradually acquiring a much more continental approach to food and living generally. I liked it and it suited me.

Was my life still in Australia? Definitely, I still had a home there. But another six months in Treviso was an experience I wanted to repeat and, as I said, in my heart I knew that I was going to do it as soon as the offer of a second season was made.

As for Isabella being a motivation for me to go back, all I can say is that there was something about her in the back of my mind that wouldn't go away. The thought of seeing her in person again gave me butterflies—'I wonder how all this will play out?' I'd had girlfriends in the past, sure, but nothing serious. Being around Isabella, even in the very early stages of courtship, seemed to give me a confidence I'd never had before. But in actual romantic terms there was technically nothing between us at this point. The pleasant exchange of letters, our friendly conversations before I left after the first season and the fact that our meetings had all been so fleeting combined to make me both curious and optimistic.

What made things a little tricky was the fact that Isabella's mother, Daniela, preferred me to Isabella's boyfriend, who was still on the scene. That was good news. But the downside was that a girl who's told what to do, or *who* to be with, by her parents usually resists and does exactly the opposite. I needed Isabella to be the exception to that rule. I needed to be persistent, but I also needed to play it pretty cool.

In the end it came down to the old 'Can you help me with my Italian?' routine (I tried everything, trust me) and that's when we started seeing each other properly.

TIM HORAN: My wife and I and our daughter, Lucy, went to stay with Noddy in Treviso after the end of the Wales and Ireland tour. We were supposed to stay at his place for four nights but we were chased out of the place after just two because Lucy was crying at night, crying in the morning and Noddy wasn't used to it! One night I accompanied him to meet Isabella at a big tennis party. She was very busy with the organising and Michael didn't quite get stood up, but he definitely got the shits a little and left after a couple of hours. When he jumped in his car, he reversed into a tree and then blamed me for it!

Life carried on with Benetton as if I'd never been away. I was enjoying being back with my teammates, we were playing good rugby and I had a new relationship that made me very happy. Part of the arrangement with the rugby club was that they arranged my accommodation each year. The place they gave me was a little studio right in the middle of town—I could literally walk out my front door into the piazza. It was pretty nice and interesting being in the historic centre of town—but it wasn't very spacious.

I remember Timmy Horan and his wife came straight from the UK tour to stay with me for a while. They'd just had a daughter and, as I now know, babies cry—particularly at night. 'Helmet' likes to say that I kicked him out, but that didn't happen. Where else was he going to go? He had nowhere else to go.

I just said, 'Mate, I'm not used to this. I'm going to use the earplugs the airline gave me.'

And that's what I did.

Another day Timmy wanted to go on a day-trip. 'Let's go to Venice!' I asked a friend of mine, Francesco Cosulich, if he wouldn't mind being a tour guide. Of course he was excited to meet Timmy, so he agreed. When we arrived in Venice and met up with Francesco, Helmet looked around and said, 'Mate, it must have been raining a lot here. All the roads are flooded!'

I don't think he was joking.

Francesco had booked us in for lunch at a very expensive restaurant called Harry's Bar. When we got there, Timmy said to me, 'I fancy pie and mash today.'

Francesco looked at me and said, 'What is pie?'

I just rolled my eyes.

Francesco said, 'It's going to be a long day!'

AFTER PLAYING WELL IN Italy for a second season, I checked in for a double hernia operation in Australia after returning from

Europe in April 1993. I'd been having niggling problems with it; it was gradually getting worse. During the World Cup Sevens in Edinburgh in March, it had started feeling considerably more painful. The operation was something I'd probably needed for a while, but I'd never quite found the right moment.

In the course of the surgery, the doctors took a couple of lymph node biopsies from my groin area for testing. When they were in there repairing the hernia, they'd seen something that looked suspicious. They were pretty concerned about it for a while but, thankfully, everything turned out to be benign. I was inactive for maybe three weeks in total.

As preparation for a one-off Test against the All Blacks in Dunedin—followed by Tests against South Africa shortly afterwards—I played first in a Test against Tonga at Ballymore and then in a club game for University against Sunnybank. I felt fine; I just needed a bit of match-time to test the groin. During that second game I got a fingernail scratch on my arm. It didn't seem like much; it was the length of a dollar coin, maybe not even that big. I thought nothing particularly of it at the time.

The following day, while I was on a flight down to Sydney to join the rest of the team prior to us leaving for the Bledisloe Cup match in Dunedin, I started to feel ill. At first I thought, 'Ah shit, I'm getting the flu.' When I got to Sydney, I went to see Cam Osborne, the Queensland doctor who was due to go to Dunedin with us, and he told me that there were a couple of other guys suffering from similar flu symptoms. I didn't train that day and was told to go to bed in the hotel. We were staying in Camperdown.

As I was lying on the bed, I remember becoming incredibly sick, to the point where I couldn't even move. I thought,

'Something's really not good.' I managed to call the hotel reception and say, 'I think I might need a bit of help here.' It was that bad. I couldn't even get to the door of my room. So they came up, opened the door, took me to the doctor and he took one look at me and said, 'You're in trouble.' Luckily, the hotel was across the road from a hospital. I was admitted and diagnosed with peritonitis. Twenty years earlier, people regularly died from peritonitis. It was beyond painful.

That whole next week wasn't good. I think I lost eight or nine kilos—a lot of weight for somebody who was pretty fit. Apparently, bacteria had entered my body via the fingernail scratch on my arm—probably as a result of contact with dirt on the ground. From there it had travelled downwards and found the area in my groin where the lymph nodes had been weakened at the time of the surgery.

The team left for Dunedin and played New Zealand with Pat Howard in my place. I missed the remainder of the summer and didn't appear again until the tour of Canada, the USA and France.

BEING TEMPORARILY RELIEVED OF goal-kicking duties has had a significant effect on my overall play on a few occasions. One example that I remember particularly well was on the tour of France during the Australian summer of 1993. Having missed South Africa's tour in Australia due to the peritonitis, I was straight back in as captain of the Test team for the French tour that stopped off for games in the USA and Canada on the way.

It was a two-Test series in France and we narrowly lost the first, 16–13, in Bordeaux. We didn't play particularly well. We had a few defensive issues and the French backs exploited them. I had a long kick to tie the match, way out on the left touchline—probably 55 metres from the posts. That's right on the end of most goal-kickers' range and probably outside mine. I missed it. I struck it really solidly—no complaints at all—I just couldn't get it there. But it wasn't one of those misses that haunted me. I never thought, 'That's one that got away.' I prepared, executed but just couldn't get it there. That happens. It wasn't like Eden Park.

The second Test was in Paris at the old Parc des Princes. It was one of those great occasions when lots of people who were close to me converged on one place. It was almost as if they *knew* they should be there. Isabella was there—it was the only time she ever saw me play for Australia in person. Her parents were there too, my dad was there, my great friend David Coe was there—it was a nice feeling to have so much support.

Bob Dwyer decided that it might be an idea if I didn't kick goals that day. I think it was partly a tactical decision to give us a few more attacking options. Campo, Timmy and Jason Little were obvious attacking threats and we all felt that there might be an opportunity to use me in a slightly more attacking role in an attempt to move the big, but not overly mobile, French back row around.

I also think that Bob recognised how much weight *not* goal-kicking might relieve me of. Marty Roebuck would take over. Bob's plan worked to perfection. If you look at the stats, you won't see my name associated with any of the points we scored in a 24–3 victory. What the stats don't say is that it was probably my best running performance in a Wallaby jersey.

With no kicking to worry about (and Marty kicked everything he looked at that day) I felt incredibly free. A gap opened; I went through it. A defender came at me; I stepped inside him. The French back-row forwards chased shadows all afternoon. *My* shadow mainly. It felt great to show what I could do as an attacking flyhalf, and to have my future wife and family there to see it only made the win sweeter.

BOB DWYER: We always thought that Michael subjected himself to self-analysis too much. In some ways it restricted him. He wanted so much not to make a wrong decision that he removed a number of potentially good ones from his repertoire. We were a better team than France in 1993. Losing the first Test was incomprehensible to me. So then we played them in Paris, which is a traditionally much more difficult place to win. Michael was already planning to end his career after 1995; we'd discussed it. I thought, 'I don't really want him to end his career without showing the French the full level of his ability.' I thought that goal-kicking imposed a number of restrictions on his performance, so I said, 'I don't want you to kick for goal.' He said, 'Why not?' I said, 'I want you to show people what you are capable of in an attacking sense.' He said, 'Righto', and then he tore France apart. Afterwards the French media said to me, 'So, this is a new Michael Lynagh?' And I said, 'No, this is normal. This is his normal capacity.' And it was.

We had a great night all together in Paris after the game. We were in one of those typically French places where they serve dinner and then, at about midnight, they move all the tables back and it becomes a nightclub. It was a really chic place to be. There were people like Yannick Noah wherever you looked.

I remember Abdel Benazzi was there that night too—the French flanker. He turned up with a bunch of the other French guys, carrying this great methuselah of champagne. When he saw me, he ran across the club, grabbed me and said, 'This is the first time I've been able to get you all day.'

TEN

A RUGBY REVOLUTION

PRIOR TO THE 1995 World Cup in South Africa, the debate about members of the squad being based somewhere other than Australia was reignited. Campo's approach wasn't helpful, just as it hadn't been back in 1992 when the debate first flared up.

A background issue was that the Australian Rugby Union had been in an awkward position for a few years over the level of control it had over the players. There were no meaningful contracts at this stage, so, as the game still wasn't professional and nobody was being paid, the Union really had very little control over what we did. In the past we'd been given a tacit message that essentially said, 'You can go where you want and do whatever kind of promotional work you like.' But at the same time we were given a list of the ARU's affiliates and told not to do anything in competition with those entities. The Union technically didn't have control of the players, but at the same time it was trying to dictate what we could and could not do.

I'd been on the wrong end of that scenario a few years earlier when I'd been approached by Power's Brewery to do an ad for them, even though Castlemaine Perkins was one of the Australian Rugby Union's (and Queensland's) main sponsors. Prior to that, I had requested a contract from the Union and it wasn't forthcoming, so I thought, 'I'll just go and do it.' I did— and it caused a controversy.

I'd taken a stand. I understood why the Union felt it had been caught on the hop when one of its star players appeared in a commercial for the rival of one of its main sponsors. But at the same time, I felt that, in the absence of a contract, it was something I was perfectly within my rights to do. In the end it was resolved when the Australian Rugby Union told me they'd ban me if I didn't stop promoting Power's, but it was indicative of the uncertainty concerning just what level of control the Union had over amateur players. Playing for clubs overseas was just one aspect of the wider issue that continued to crop up in the years immediately prior to players being paid.

All that said, from a control perspective, Campo had a point. He probably felt that if he was going to be dictated to, he should somehow be compensated. By suggesting that he'd go and play and promote himself in other countries, he was merely choosing to exercise his options, which is fair enough. We just had slightly different ways of handling things, both of them valid. My main feeling was that I loved playing for Australia and wanted to play for Australia. I felt obliged, for the love of the sport, to do what guys had been doing for a hundred years: to play for my country for the love of it, and to do so with the best interests of my teammates foremost.

Part of the problem was that, with a World Cup build-up in full swing, the Australian Rugby Union was a little uncomfortable about having a member of the squad—the *captain* of the squad, no less—living and playing in another country. From that perspective, I guess the Union had a valid point. However, I'd already signed an agreement with Benetton that took me through until after the World Cup, and I wasn't about to renege on that arrangement for the sake of a few training camps. I thought, 'I'm caught in the middle here.'

Unlike my previous three seasons in Italy, when I'd only returned to Australia once the Italian domestic championship was over, late 1994 into early 1995 was different in that the ARU had arranged five squad training camps, spaced at various intervals throughout that time period. The aim was to monitor how everyone was doing, first of all, but they were also intended to facilitate the integration of a whole new group of support staff who were now considered part of the squad. Everyone was expected to be there—no excuses.

The rationale behind this dated back to the period immediately after we won the World Cup in 1991. It was an obvious pinnacle and we'd continued to be successful for a couple of years afterwards with what was still a very good side. The game was moving forward and becoming more technical, and in response to those technical demands, Bob Dwyer (and the other major nations' coaches) jumped on the popular idea that you needed to bring in experts to advise on specific aspects of play, preparation or recovery that neither he nor we, the players, were particularly knowledgeable about.

In principle it all made sense. It was rugby evolution in action. But when we'd all get together for a training camp, a large proportion of our time seemed to be taken up by the various focus sessions with the new experts. In the past, we'd just trained.

Now, the dietician might want her hour here, and the weights trainer his hour there—all these people wanted time with the team, and justifiably so. After all, if I'd been employed by the Australian Rugby Union to talk to the team and be the designated dietician or psychologist or whatever, I'd want to stamp my influence on the team; my reputation would be on the line. I understood that. But I worried that if the support staff's expectations weren't managed properly, there was a real risk of a situation where we were trying to run before we could walk.

From the time the squad training camp issue was first raised, at no point did I think, 'Well, screw you, guys. I'm staying put in Italy because my fiancée is here.' (Isabella and I had got engaged a few months earlier.) I was the captain of the team and I never adopted a confrontational stance at any point. The role meant a lot to me. I led by example and I would lead by example going forward. It wasn't as if I had ever disappeared to Italy and said, 'Okay folks, see you next year.' I was always in touch with both the Queensland and the international selectors when I was in Italy, keeping myself in the equation by playing fair with them, and setting a good example to the younger Wallaby players by being an integral part of the squad. The bottom line was that my commitment was not going to be in any way influenced by where I was living or playing.

In the end, the ARU saved me from having to initiate what would have been an embarrassing 'You know that agreement I just signed? Well, I'm going to have to back out of it' conversation with Benetton. They agreed that I could stay in Italy, on the condition that I kept in close contact with the coaches and returned for some of the squad weekends.

On that front they perhaps underestimated me. I took it upon myself to send regular videotapes of my matches back from Italy to the coaches. Not just that, I flew back for *all* the training weekends. I paid for the flights out of my own pocket. I didn't complain about it, nor did I do it for show. Did I have jetlag? Of course I did. But I wanted to demonstrate, via my actions, that I was part of the squad and that as captain I'd do anything required to lead by example. Not just that, I wanted to be there to be part of the team spirit.

In the end it worked out okay. The trips were constructive from a 'let's get everyone together' standpoint. That part was really worthwhile. Isabella even came with me for one of the camps. But the issue I still had was with the structuring of the camp sessions, now that we had several extra staff kicking their heels on the touchline. I was wary of this before we even got to the World Cup.

WHEN WE GOT TO South Africa for the 1995 World Cup, the general atmosphere had ramped up significantly from what we'd experienced three years earlier. While it had been a great, if at times a little scary, atmosphere in 1992, the interest in the game had been largely confined to the white population. While the black population was supportive of us Wallabies, as I recall, and mildly interested in the concept of touring rugby teams, there was a sense that apartheid wasn't far enough in the country's rear-view mirror for them to feel truly included in all the excitement.

By 1995, all that had changed. Nelson Mandela's charisma seemed to have had a unifying effect in the intervening three years and that meant that the entire country was massively excited about the prospect of a World Cup where the home nation seemed to have an excellent chance of winning the tournament.

I really noticed the difference. The population felt like this powerful sixteenth man. And that's before we even set foot on a rugby pitch. We were the reigning World Champions and all eyes were on us. With hindsight, I'm not sure that we wore the mantle particularly well.

When you're in the spotlight, part of you wants to hide, whereas another part of you quite likes it. It's entirely natural. I wouldn't call it arrogance, but I'd be lying if I said that there wasn't just a little bit of over-confidence around that squad, although I wasn't conscious of it at the time. You try not to believe the hype around being the defending champions, but as hard as you try to push hubris away, when you're the World Cup holders I don't think you ever fully shake it off.

SEAN FITZPATRICK, FORMER ALL BLACK CAPTAIN: After we won the World Cup in 1987, we turned up in 1991 with a bit of complacency. We were wandering around London in black coats, not talking to anyone, thinking we were pretty cool. A bit fat, a bit lazy, and it seemed to me that the Wallabies were in a similar frame of mind in South Africa. I remember seeing them arrive somewhere in their tour bus, all wearing sunglasses and thinking they were pretty special. I remember saying to Phil Kearns, 'You guys think you're better than what you are—look at you with your sunglasses.' I recognised that immediately because, as former World Cup winners, we'd been there. Australia was there for the picking—too many of them were a bit long in the tooth.

I had basic concerns about our preparation. First, and I've thought about this a million times since, I always felt we spent far too long in South Africa prior to the tournament. I'm all for acclimatising—getting there, shaking off the stiffness, the jetlag, getting a feel for the lie of the land, but it seemed we took it way too far by arriving a full ten days in advance of our first group match against South Africa at Newlands on May 25th.

It probably sounds like a petty thing, but I think that when you're trying to peak for a sporting event, it pays to be fresh and energised when the whistle blows, rather than feeling bored and stale. Don't get me wrong, Bob's idea of getting to South Africa in time to acclimatise and prepare was okay in principle, but I think we took it a bit far. We were like a boxer who's ready for a fight. He's been training for months, waiting for the bell to ring. He wants to arrive at the venue, go to the dressing room, get taped up, get his gloves on—and then all he wants to do is fight. He doesn't want to be sitting in that dressing room, days in advance, tired, bored and on a downwards track in terms of physical and mental sharpness.

So there was that, and, as I mentioned earlier, by the summer of 1995 the culture of getting specialist coaches involved in every aspect of the game was very much part of world rugby. Everyone was doing it. Dieticians, psychologists, physiologists, weight trainers, backs coaches, forwards coaches—you name it, they were all on board.

SEAN FITZPATRICK: We were adding support staff to the squad but to a much lesser degree. Australian sport in the late '80s and early '90s was on a high and they were really pushing the envelope more than anyone else. They were by far the best rugby team in the world in 1991. That continued in 1992. They were pushing the envelope, but we were doing things that our Union just wasn't paying for. Zinzan Brooke and I had to pay for our own trainer. We were using Swiss balls and our coach would say, 'What the hell is that? Get that out of here ...'

As an interesting reference point, I often thought about 1984. We had thirty-two players for the nineteen-match Grand Slam tour, plus a coach, a manager, a forwards coach and a doctor. Four support staff; that was it. It really was changed days. Somebody told me recently that when England tour nowadays, there are two support staff for every player. So for a thirty-man touring party, there would be sixty staff tending to every aspect of getting the players ready for a game.

ROB ANDREW, FORMER ENGLAND FLYHALF: I always felt that the period between 1991 and 1995 was the build-up to the professional game. In fact it was pretty clear after the 1991 World Cup that— at some point in the very near future—the game was going to go professional. It was more and more coaches, more and more commitment to training, more preparation time. We had more and more staff by 1995; that's just the way the game was going. We had forwards coach, backs coach, head coach, kicking coach, more and more support staff. Not like they have today, but a lot more than we had in the '80s. You felt like you were heading towards being a full-time player.

In retrospect, it might also be that the 1995 World Cup represented the end of a cycle for Australian rugby. I always think that five years is about the natural lifespan of a rugby coach anyway, particularly when he's got more or less the same players to work with in those years. There is a definite shelf life. Very rarely in rugby do you see a Sir Alex Ferguson, an Arsène Wenger. Guy Novès, who's been the coach at Toulouse for over twenty years, is the exception.

Beyond five years I always think that—certainly at national level—there's a risk of the coach–team relationship becoming a bit jaded. That's not a criticism. It's just that, by that point, the team has heard all the coach's ideas. Eventually, nobody talks and nobody listens. It's like a marriage in its final throes. That's how it had worked with Alan Jones, who took us from before the Grand Slam tour in 1984 through the World Cup in 1987. As fantastic a man and coach as Alan Jones was and still is, he had nothing left to give. The relationship had run its natural course.

But when Bob Dwyer came back to the team in 1988 for his second spell in charge, it was as if the imprint of his first tenure had been erased. Any fantastic results he'd achieved still stood, of course, but his old habits had gone and even if some remained he had a new set of players to work with who didn't know them anyway.

Bob had matured a lot as a coach since his first stint from 1982 to '83. The game had moved on—so had he, and to his credit, there's no doubt that he was a lot more thorough when it came to preparation than he'd ever been back in the early 1980s. The evolution of the game demanded that.

Back in 1983, Bob had been very old school in his rugby ideas, although in fairness to him he was probably a little less old school than many of his contemporaries. But by the time his second tenure came around (after we'd been knocked out of the World Cup in '87), he had become much more interested in training methods and preparation. You had to be, or you simply didn't survive.

Bob also had become very adept at finding the right balance within a team—that important blend of youth, experience and the intangibles. Campo, for example, wasn't always the easiest to manage. He sought attention sometimes, as if his brilliance on the field didn't bring him enough of it. You had to be strong with him without either alienating him or letting him enforce his wishes on the team as a whole. Bob knew how to handle him personally and how to extricate the most out of him as a player. He knew how to manage all of us, and that was quite a skill to have. You could call it synergy, and he really made it work.

Yes, he had some problems in the first couple of years when he came back: 1988 and '89 were poor years by our standards, but he was rebuilding. You have to build to get to the top. Set some goals. Measure your progress. Then, in 1991, everything clicked. Australia had that perfect storm of the right players at the right stages of their careers overseen by the coach who knew how to get the best out of them.

Anyway, you could say that we were on the right track in that we had all become much more knowledgeable about specific areas of the game and preparation, but I think we took the approach too far, too quickly and perhaps didn't quite manage it properly—to the point where we possibly lost sight of the bigger picture.

In theory, Bob's focus on the consultants was absolutely right. But there were two sides to the implementation. Bob had to first identify the need for the consultants in our system. He'd done that, and we'd had a small window of opportunity to bed them in prior to the World Cup. But it was also vitally important that he managed their various expectations within the squad set-up. Yes, they were on board and part of the new direction, but the players' freshness and physical wellbeing still had to be the number one priority, in my opinion. It was a question of emphasis and I looked at it and thought, 'I don't envy Bob here. This is not an easy balance.'

BOB DWYER: I've tried to think about it without getting too upset, seeing as it's in the past. In my mind, there was definitely a possibility—or even a probability—that paralysis by over-analysis played a part [in Australia's elimination in the quarter-finals of the World Cup]. Subconsciously, maybe there was a bit of complacency too—people thinking more about outcomes than actual performance. Frequently, when trying to move forward, one sometimes goes in the wrong direction. You need to keep moving, but in an effort to move, you need to remember what the destination is. Also, and I've thought about it a lot: if the sports psychologist is doing his job, he should not be at the competition venue. His role should be to teach skills which the player himself takes forward, not to be there acting as a prop. In 1995, he was there as a prop.

From a captain and player's perspective, the primary practical downside for us was that we had too many meetings. Rugby players train, run, kick and then run some more. That's what we do. I'm not suggesting that we shouldn't then come off the paddock, sit down and say, 'That was good, that wasn't, he was good, he was crap.' That would have been fine. But these were long meetings with lots of talking, lots of deep analysis—they were much more like a finance or business seminar than a rugby team's preparation.

Then we combined these long meetings with getting on the training field and staying there far too long. Sometimes a training session would be three hours or more—far longer than any game or even any *two* games. I was always one for the old-school approach of training very hard for a solid hour. Emptying everything out, breathing hard—feeling like you've really exerted yourself. Then coming off for a rest, saying, 'That was a great, hard session. That worked well, that didn't work, let's try this tomorrow, let's never do that again.' Instead, all we felt at the end was 'Jeez, that lasted forever but we could have done so much better in a focused shorter session.'

I'd always enjoyed practising and developing my skills at full speed to simulate a match situation, not training at half-pace. You had it planned, everyone knew exactly what they were doing, and you were done in an hour. That's what most of us were used to. Suddenly we found ourselves standing around on the training field not doing very much of anything. It didn't feel as if we were *achieving* enough.

Also, once we knew that we were likely to be out in the Cape Town sun for three hours, we paced ourselves for the first hour of training, simply because we didn't know what was coming later. I'd think to myself, 'What if the last hour of three is a fitness session?' I kept a bit in reserve just in case. Anyone sensible would have done the same thing. The problem was, I think we ended up playing like that on the pitch too. Your body becomes conditioned to saving something because that's what you've done in training. And you can't keep anything for yourself in international rugby. You can only focus on what's in front of you there and then. You live for that day and that day only. And if you get injured or are too drained to come out and do it the next day, the squad is there specifically to provide back-up and someone else can be brought in. That's how it should be.

IT'S HARD TO OVERSTATE just how important that opening match with South Africa was for both teams. It wasn't just a huge rugby match—it was a momentous spectacle, especially given the hype and expectation that was being piled on the hosts. Playing the defending World Champions was a monumental national occasion for the host nation, but in simple rugby terms—and this is the only part I tried to focus on—the game would decide which side of the draw you were on. We'd need to take small steps, successfully, to achieve our goal.

It was pretty easy to work out. If we lost, and the other pool games went on form, we would more than likely play New Zealand in the semis—a side that any team wanted to avoid until the final. Admittedly, the All Blacks hadn't had a great 1994 season. Unusually, they were slightly understated—they might even have been trying to fly under the radar. But with the likes of Jonah Lomu on the wing needing six people to tackle him, there was only so far under the radar they could fly.

On the other hand, win the South African game and we'd go the other route, with a kinder draw that, on paper, looked as if it would lead to a semi-final against the perennially unpredictable French in Durban. We knew very well what the French were capable of, but we weren't even thinking about them. Our aim, like everyone else's, was to win the World Cup. The first step was finding a way to beat the hosts.

In the few days prior to the game, we kept seeing pictures of the South African players in the papers, and one of them really grabbed me. I was having breakfast with Bob Dwyer and prominent in that morning's paper was a shot of the Springboks training. It almost seemed like sporting propaganda, put out there to get in our heads. The players were running with their shirts off, and when I saw it, I said to myself, 'Oh my God. They look pretty lean, these boys.' I thought of myself as being pretty fit, but you wouldn't have persuaded me to take my shirt off for a photograph, I can assure you. The Springboks had serious muscles, six-packs etc. They looked ready. Then there were the reports of the very strict diet they were subjected to: mainly rice and boiled chicken. We had that as part of our regimen too, but judging by the pictures, they'd had a lot less of it.

As if nagging doubts about our preparation weren't distraction enough, there was a background issue that did me no favours prior to the first game against South Africa. I was made aware, in my capacity as the captain of Australia, of a proposed professional rugby breakaway competition, to be run by the so-called World Rugby Corporation (WRC for short), just before one of the biggest games of my life. It would have been huge news whenever I heard it, but the timing could hardly have been worse.

The conversation came about almost by accident. On the Thursday before the Saturday match, I asked for a meeting with Bob. I felt the need for us to sit down, captain to coach— to make sure we were both on the same page. I wanted to ask

Playing cricket for a Queensland Juniors side on tour in New South Wales. I was twelve or thirteen and I think I made a few runs that day.

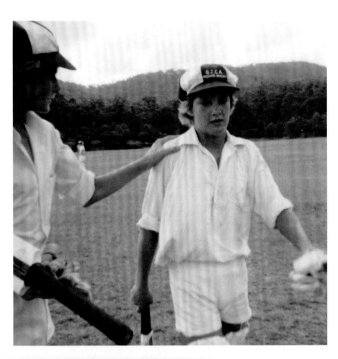

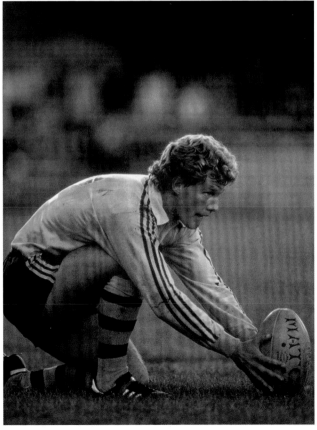

Lining up another three points, I hope, during the 1984 Grand Slam Tour.

Getty Images

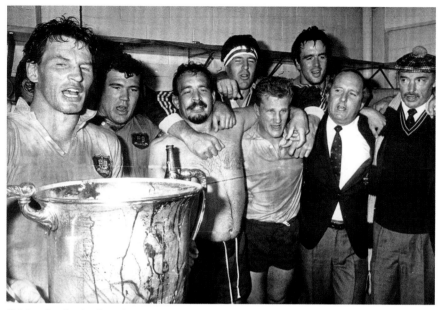

Celebrating in the dressing room at Eden Park, Auckland, after we beat New Zealand 22–9 to win the 1986 Bledisloe Cup. No Australian team has repeated the feat in New Zealand since. Left to right: Simon Poidevin, Tom Lawton, Enrique 'Topo' Rodriguez, Ross Reynolds, me, Steve Cutler, coach Alan Jones and our forwards coach Alec Evans. *Ross Setford*

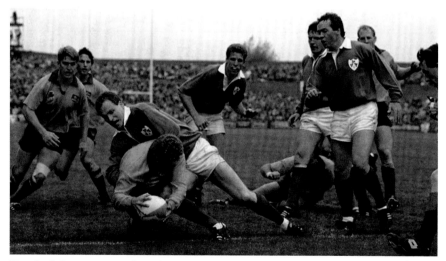

The single best moment of my playing career and the try that shattered the dreams of a nation! Going over in the corner with minutes remaining in the 1991 World Cup quarter-final against Ireland. *Press Association Images*

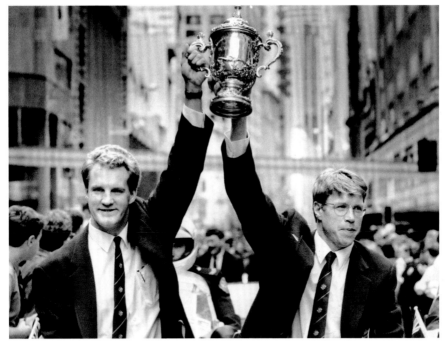

When we were told there was to be a parade in Sydney to celebrate our winning the 1991 World Cup, I thought, 'God, I hope a few people turn up.' But when we got there, we were shocked by the size of the crowd that came out to greet us with the trophy.

Fairfax/Craig Golding

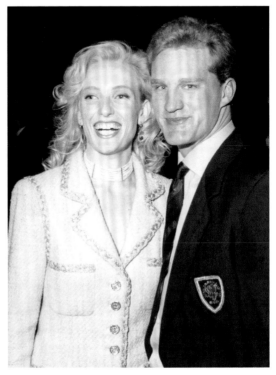

My wife Isabella and me at the Benetton Treviso Christmas party in 1993.

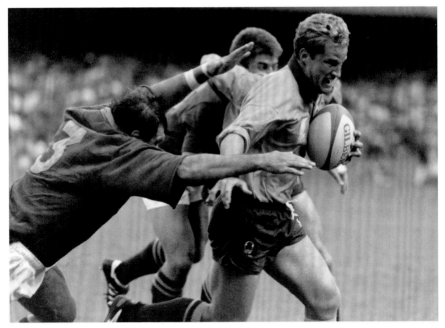

Trying to avoid a few South Africans on my way to scoring the first try of the 1995 World Cup at Newlands. *Author's collection*

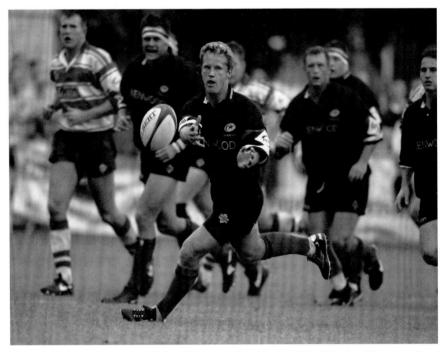

Playing for Saracens against Sale at Heywood Road in the Allied Dunbar Premiership One match in 1997. We won 19–10. *David Rogers/Allsport/Getty*

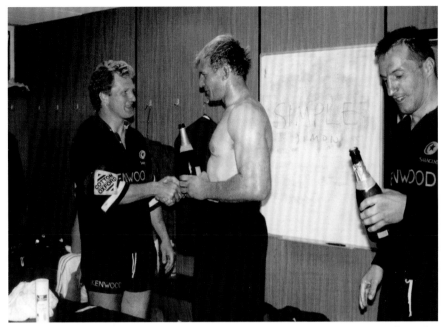

In the dressing room after my last competitive game in 1998. Francois Pienaar (centre) and Philippe Sella (right) are opening the champagne. *Author's collection*

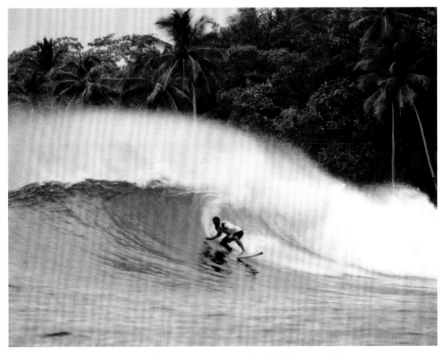

One of my great loves in life. Catching a wave in the Maldives in 2008.

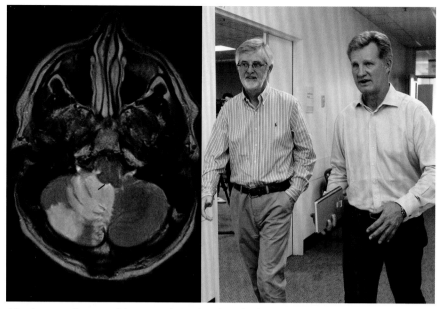

A brain scan shows a white area about the size of a fist on the bottom left. This is the area of stroke in the right, rear part of my brain. The small black line indicates where the swollen cerebellum is very close to coming into contact with my brain stem. The consequences would have been devastating. Right: My father Ian and me leaving the press conference at the Royal Brisbane and Women's Hospital. In my right hand I have the notebook I used to write down my thoughts while I was in hospital. *Glenn Barnes/Newspix*

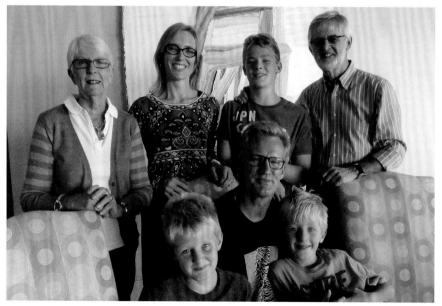

The morning of my fiftieth birthday in Cape Town. Back (left to right): My mother Marie, Isabella, my eldest Louis and my father Ian. Front (left to right): My middle son Thomas, me, and my youngest son Nicolo.

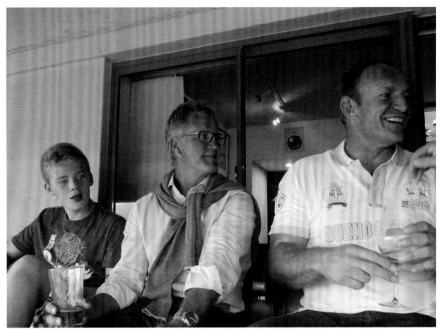

Watching the 2013 Currie Cup Final at Newlands between Western Province and Natal with my son Louis and friend and former Saracens teammate Francois Pienaar.

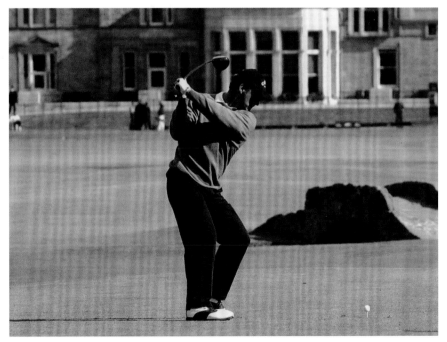

Another great sporting love of mine. Teeing off at the eighteenth hole at St Andrews in the Alfred Dunhill Links Championship in 2003. *Author's collection*

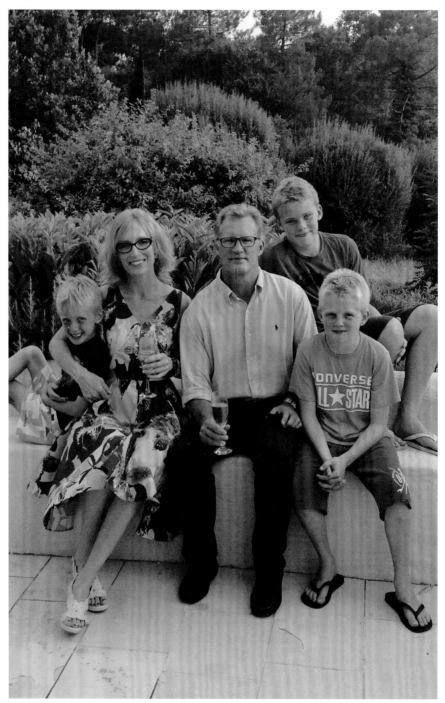

The Lynagh family on holiday in Bidart, France, in 2013.

'How are we doing as a squad?' and, just as importantly, 'How am *I* doing?'

It felt like we'd hardly had a conversation since we'd arrived in South Africa. My teammates were on my back about the time we were spending on the training pitch, and it was my role as their captain to listen and to pass the comments on. I needed to talk to Bob and find a way to streamline the sessions a bit. It made sense to me to wind things down. The matches were imminent. Big matches. I thought we should taper proceedings a little to keep the guys fresh. I thought I could pitch the idea pretty convincingly.

So Bob and I met and sat outside another hotel one afternoon after training. We were chatting away, having a cup of tea in the sunshine. He saw my point of view about the training set-up. He agreed with me on the whole but was wary about upsetting the squad atmosphere as far as the support staff were concerned. At least he was listening, though. I could go back to the guys and say, 'Look, I've asked if we can condense the sessions.' They'd understand the position I was in, and once the matches began I was sure it would be less of an issue anyway.

'Look, Nod, there's another thing I wanted to talk to you about ...'

I put my cup down.

'Yeah? What's that?'

And with that Bob went on to outline this planned breakaway rugby idea, reminiscent of what Kerry Packer had done with cricket in the late 1970s. It, involved us, New Zealand, South Africa and the Home Nations breaking away from the International Rugby Board to form a new, televised rugby competition. It was seemingly still very hush-hush, as I obviously knew nothing about it. I hadn't seen it coming at all.

BOB DWYER: I think there was, initially at least, less talk about the breakaway in our squad than in others. Not many of the Wallaby team even knew about it. Only the guys who'd been approached by rugby league knew about it. But it was me who told Michael because he'd already mentioned to me that he was planning to retire.

The details were sketchy. At that stage nobody really knew who the backers were or exactly what was on the table. There was big talk—but *only* talk—of A$150,000 a year contracts and the like, which, given that we were earning nothing at the time, was obviously very significant money.

Bob said, 'We should be telling all the team this.'

'Well no, we shouldn't be.'

I respected Bob's opinion, but I thought the timing was terrible. I felt that it would be a distraction the team didn't need.

Sticking in my mind also was the fact that, back in Australia, there was major upheaval going on within the sport of rugby league—an upheaval that involved a few of our squad. Basically, there was a bidding war going on between the existing rugby league set-up run by the Australian Rugby League and a planned Rupert Murdoch and News Limited-backed 'Super League'.

It was the upstart News-backed guys versus the establishment. Entire teams like the Brisbane Broncos (who were owned by News Limited) had broken away completely from the traditional set-up and individual players were being asked to choose which side they wanted to go with. Big money was being thrown around as an incentive to sign and both sides of this rugby league war were also aggressively pursuing our centres, Jason Little and Tim Horan, as part of the ongoing war to attract the best players.

I knew that Timmy and Jason were considering their options. I didn't blame them. They needed to make a living like anyone else. I thought that the best thing to do would be for me to take them aside, as their captain, and give them a heads-up as to what might be down the line. I did that, but didn't share all of the information I was privy to at that stage. I felt that to start throwing numbers around—numbers that sounded like they'd been plucked from thin air anyway— would only be unsettling and counterproductive in a squad context. All Timmy and Jason needed to know was that there were alternatives on the horizon in rugby union and therefore they shouldn't hastily commit to rugby league as the only financially attractive option. I felt that they needed some basic information so that they could make educated decisions after the World Cup. As friends, I only wanted the best for them.

Also, while the breakaway wasn't quite the talk of the tournament, I was pretty certain that Francois Pienaar and Sean Fitzpatrick at the very least knew as much as I did. From a trust perspective I wanted the information to come from me, their captain, not from somebody outside the Australian camp. I didn't want Timmy and Jason to feel that I'd withheld information from them that was crucial to their future. I'd played with them too long, we'd come this far, and I respected them both far too much to be in any way underhand.

SEAN FITZPATRICK: We knew nothing about it until after the final. On the Sunday morning after the final, we were invited to go round to somebody's house and that's where we were told. Some of the guys that weren't playing in the final had been approached on the previous Friday, but other than that we knew nothing. It probably epitomised our standing in world rugby at that time. We were not the number-one ranked team in 1994 and 1995, although they obviously needed the All Blacks to go. We just weren't the reigning World Champions.

TIM HORAN: Even before the World Cup, Jason and I had had a combined offer to go to a couple of different clubs involved in the Super League breakaway, and so the first person we confided in was Noddy. It didn't affect our concentration on the World Cup, but it just let him know what was going on. Equally, he kept us informed about the potential the WRC could have once the World Cup was over. He basically said, 'Hold your horses until after the tournament.'

Predictably, given what was at stake, the breakaway issue escalated significantly as the tournament went along and at one point I was offered a significant amount of money—A$250,000 to be precise—to basically 'deliver' my team to the organisers on a plate. They requested a letter of intent from all the players. In addition, I was to be offered a contract, but as I'd decided that I was retiring after the World Cup anyway, that part didn't concern me.

I said, 'Look, I don't want to get involved with all this at the moment. But I want to be kept in the picture as to what's going on.'

The organisers said: 'Okay, we'll do that.'

I *was* kept in the picture as things developed. But at the same time I was adamant that I didn't want my team side-tracked by this chatter, apart from the guys I'd already told. So I gathered information as the tournament progressed and kept most of it to myself. I knew that was the policy that would give the team the best chance in the World Cup.

It might surprise you if I told you that I don't remember many specific details about the games in that World Cup—but I've never really remembered all the ins and outs of any game. Even directly after a game, sitting in the changing room, heart still pounding, I wouldn't remember too much. I was always— as coaches and psychologists like to call it—'in the moment'. I think that's a compliment. Then I'd move on to the next moment and the next and it would take me a while after the game to piece all these components together. Sometimes I never reconciled them at all.

BOB DWYER: Looking back on that first game I think, 'Maybe we over-trained—maybe we should have tapered things off a bit earlier.'

After what seemed like an endless build-up, South Africa came out very organised, very well coached and extremely well captained on that May 25th afternoon at Newlands in Cape Town. On paper it was close and on the pitch it was too. On reflection, in my position as captain, it was also the single tensest encounter I've ever been involved in.

I remember looking around at some of the younger guys and thinking, 'Jeez, you look pretty overawed by this.' And

I didn't blame them. After all, I—a guy who'd been around the block a few times and had seen pretty much everything—struggled to cope with the huge partisan crowd and the sense of history. What chance did these young guys have? What chance did *any* of us have?

It was a big, big occasion and one that South Africa at home, in their first ever World Cup game, definitely dealt with better than we did. We didn't play like World Champions; we played like a group of guys who'd forgotten what the aim of the game actually was.

We were slow, rigid and devoid of ideas. South Africa were keen, hungry and ready to remove the decades of exile-sized chip from their shoulders at our expense. Defeat, albeit a narrower one than we warranted, meant that our route through the tournament was decided. We'd get the All Blacks in the semis.

If we even got there.

ROB ANDREW: Although none of us would have admitted it at the time, the Australia game carried a fair bit of payback for our defeat in the 1991 World Cup final. We'd been beaten at home, at Twickenham, and a lot of the same players were still involved, on both sides. My overriding memory is that it was a cat-and-mouse game that became a kicking contest. Michael and I traded kicks. That's how it went. Pressure kicks all the way through.

The game against England in the quarter-final is one that I don't remember too much about. I think I've mentally blanked out more of that one than some others. In hindsight it was a misjudgement, but beforehand I felt, 'It's England and we should have the beating of them.'

Saying that, I do remember just enough in general terms to say that we weren't great at all. It still felt as if we had no new ideas. We lacked attacking direction and, fortunately, England did too. Still, we somehow managed one try each. At least we had each other's moves covered from a defensive standpoint. It was a stalemate. I remember thinking, 'If we can hang in there, maybe I can make this a kicking contest between me and Rob Andrew.' That seemed like our best chance of winning.

Those are just vague, hazy recollections. And I must have been a clairvoyant, because the kicking contest part came true. He kicked one; I kicked one. Then he kicked one and then I didn't. I never got another chance. It was quite straightforward really: we lost 25–22.

One strange memory that did stay with me, though, was something very specific and also rather delicate—not a word that you'd normally associate with a World Cup quarter-final. I remember the sensation of air brushing past my hand as Rob Andrew's match-winning drop goal headed towards the posts. I rarely get a moment to step back and look at the beauty or romance in someone else's work. This would have been quite pretty to watch, if it hadn't knocked us out.

In my role as his on-rushing opposite number, I knew exactly what he was going to do. But knowing that and doing something about it were two different things.

The sequence played out in slow motion. As Rob kicked, I was close to him but not close enough. I often wish that I'd just touched the ball a little bit to divert it off course, but no—I didn't get there. Instead I was powerless—a mere spectator watching the final act of my international career playing out. I saw the maker's name on the ball quite clearly—Gilbert—but

I couldn't stop it going past me. All I felt was the Newlands air. All I thought was, 'Well, you did ask for a kicking contest ...'

ROB ANDREW: It was pre-planned from the lineout. We'd won a penalty in our own half and Mike Catt—who had a long boot on him—kicked for touch. On the way to the lineout, Dewi [Morris, the England halfback] and I were discussing that we should throw to Martin Bayfield and then catch and drive to see if we could get within range so that I could have a go. So by the time I actually received the ball from the drive, I was probably standing on the ten-yard line and when I struck it I thought, 'That's *going*.' It was probably as sweet as I'd ever struck a ball. It started going towards the right-hand post and there was a little nervousness that it was going to drift, but it had the legs by a long distance. It just flew. If I hadn't got it off the ground so quickly, Michael may well have charged it down.

Then I remember turning around to look at where it was going.

'Ah, shit, that's never missing.'

I wasn't wrong. It wasn't missing. It was quite a long way out but it was still rising as it went over—never even threatening to go anywhere but over—and at that moment I knew two things: (1) we were out of the World Cup and (2) I'd played my last match for Australia.

BOB DWYER: We were as good as England. In fact, I left my seat in the stand and came down to the sideline to prepare for extra time. Then Rob Andrew kicked the field goal that gave England the win.

ELEVEN

RETIREMENT

I'D ALREADY DECIDED THAT the 1995 World Cup would be the
end of my international career, whether we won it or not. I
hadn't officially announced it in advance. I'd only mentioned it
quietly to Bob Dwyer. It was a gut decision and I knew—and
still do know—it was the right one. I had no regrets whatsoever.
England just happened to be my last game.

I'd been on the scene for my country for twelve years and
that seemed like a pretty good innings. I'd played well, enjoyed
it and had a legacy that I was extremely proud of. I felt powerful
saying to myself, 'This is it.' Of course it would have been nice
to go out with a World Cup win as captain, but when I think
about it honestly, beaten quarter-finalists was about our level
in 1995.

It's worth adding that I'm sure we weren't alone in having
some difficulty adjusting to the rapid expansion of support staff
at the time. I'd be amazed if New Zealand and South Africa,
at least, weren't implementing similar programs. Maybe they
were a little bit better at it. And maybe they were simply better

teams and we just weren't good enough to go any further. Still, in moments of deep, but largely unfounded, optimism, I used to say to myself: 'Maybe we could have got to a semi ...'

But when I got a grip on myself and thought about it logically, the facts spoke for themselves. We'd already been beaten by South Africa. Were we better than New Zealand? Probably not. And—as disappointing as it was—we were beaten by England, who in turn were literally run over by New Zealand. Even I couldn't really argue with those stats.

Granted, we'd been carrying players who weren't one hundred per cent fit, because they were deemed to be better than the alternatives left at home. There were tough decisions to make sometimes, and the toughest questions to address are those that don't actually have an answer. For instance: 'Is Timmy Horan at eighty per cent better than Player X at one hundred per cent?' We decided that he was. Sometimes those decisions work for you.

Additionally, there were quite a few young guys for whom this was a first World Cup and, on the flip side, there were a few of us who were grimly hanging on by our fingernails, determined to enjoy one more World Cup. Were we the best people to be playing? Was I? We'll never know. But these were the kinds of questions that came up. While you consider all that, one last fact you can't avoid is that nobody has successfully defended the World Cup. Maybe there are a few lessons in that, too. It's very hard to win them back to back.

BOB DWYER: In the final analysis, we went in as favourites but didn't play as well as we could have. We'll never know all the reasons, but there's no doubt that certain players were not at their peak and that makes the difference when you're trying to win at the very highest level. If we'd been at our best, we would have beaten South Africa in the pool match. Would we have beaten them in the final? I doubt it. Would we have beaten New Zealand in the final? I would say not.

Almost as disappointing as our exit from the World Cup was the fact that I was more or less left to face the Australian media on my own. The touring party pretty much evaporated after the quarter-final. The rules of the tournament state that if you go out in the quarter-finals, you go home. If you wanted to stay on in South Africa with family or friends for a holiday, you had to pay for that yourself.

A lot of players and coaching staff stayed for the finals. Bob Dwyer stayed. The team manager, John Breen, stayed. I was the most senior member of the party who went home and that added to the disappointment. Sure, it's nice to have a holiday, see some elephants—I don't begrudge anyone that. But I definitely felt a little let down. As far as I was concerned, my flight was booked and the ticket said 'Sydney' on it.

While I don't blame people for staying and watching the final, and never said anything publicly at the time, on arriving in Sydney I was, in effect, the focal point of a losing Australian team. I saw the press gathered as I walked into the arrivals hall of the airport and I immediately felt, 'I'm out on a limb here a little.'

The press had every right to be lying in wait. We'd gone from defending champions to failures in what seemed like the blink of an eye, and I had to absorb the accompanying disappointment and answer all the questions. We'd held the

Cup; now we weren't even the fourth-best team in the world. I was there to be shot at, in a figurative sense.

Really, they should have been shooting at all of us. What could I do but deal with the press, apologise to the fans and handle it all in the only way I knew: by taking it on the chin. I said something that amounted to: 'We just weren't good enough.' And the press and fans knew me well enough to know it was true. It's always better to be upfront.

One thing I couldn't help smiling ruefully about when I was doing the post-mortems was the fact that we, Australia, had analysed the mistakes the All Blacks had made between winning the World Cup in 1987 and going out in the semi-final in '91. We logged their errors, came up with all kinds of measures and contingencies and then went and repeated most of the mistakes ourselves. When it came to it, we'd learned no lessons.

NICK FARR-JONES: I had moved to live in Paris in 1995 and was working for Société Générale. I was watching the Australian preparation from a distance. They'd had a good 1994 season, had beaten New Zealand, but something definitely went awry between 1994 and 1995. The impression I got was that it wasn't an overly harmonious team and I do know that they were distracted by the prospect of the game going professional and I think Bob [Dwyer] was very much central to that discussion.

It was a tough time and I was as disappointed as anyone. I also felt there was pressure on me from all kinds of other angles. I'd just retired from a long career playing international rugby. It's an emotional moment when you call it a day after so many years. I felt, 'I'd like to savour this a little bit, reflect on what I've done.' After all, I was actually quite content that my international career was over.

The professional rugby scenario seemed to be coming to a head. It looked like there was major upheaval about to happen and the uncertainty was unsettling, even though I'd taken myself off the table in an international sense. Of no less importance, I had a fiancée on the other side of the world. I wanted to be with her, *needed* to be with her. A huge part of my life had just drawn to a close and I wanted to share those moments. Furthermore, we had a wedding to plan, and a whole lifetime beyond that.

All these thoughts and pressures seemed suddenly to converge. I called Dad and said, 'Let's watch the semi-final somewhere.' I was staying on the Sunshine Coast so he drove up from Brisbane to meet me. As always, Dad had the right kind of advice—'You've had an amazing international career. Focus on that and what you want to do next, not anything negative in the past.' Of course, he was right.

ROB ANDREW: The Australians had obviously all gone, but at the World Cup final dinner, professional rugby was the only topic of conversation among all the players. I think, in hindsight, the general feeling has been that had they issued contracts in South Africa when they had all the players in one place, they would have got it off the ground. It was that close. The mistake they made was allowing everybody to go back home then trying to finalise things from a distance. That allowed the unions to get in to the various countries to disrupt it, which, in turn, allowed the IRB [International Rugby Board] to say, 'Okay, the game's open from

August.' My understanding is that the South Africans broke ranks first in that Francois Pienaar did a deal with their union to keep all their players tied to the SARU. Then all the other unions got their act together.

I'D EVENTUALLY SAID A conclusive 'no' to delivering the players to the World Rugby Corporation as requested. As for my retirement, did the money I could potentially earn as a professional player with WRC tempt me to hang on a bit longer? Of course it did. But the most important factor for me was that I didn't want to tarnish my whole career by being the guy who led his team into what could have been a short-lived breakaway circus.

I felt my legacy, at that point, was good. I'd played for Australia for thirteen years. Not many people can say they've done that. I didn't want to act in a way that would adversely affect the Australian Rugby Union. There was a principle there. I felt like I had bound myself to an unwritten code of loyalty, and I wasn't prepared to throw it all away. Although the ARU had never paid me anything, they'd always been extremely good to me. Of course the money incentive to break ranks was good—and who doesn't like money? But there were opportunities elsewhere that didn't involve turning my back on the ARU.

And I didn't want to be the guy who said to my Wallaby teammates, 'Come on and sign. This is the best thing for you.' I didn't want to be responsible for some of the younger guys never playing for Australia again, because it was a distinct possibility that they would be banned if they joined the breakaways. I didn't want to be the leader of that. I was happy to lead them as the captain of Australia on a rugby field, but not in a situation where I was being paid to deliver them to somebody else. These were teammates, friends and human beings—not commodities to be traded for cash. I walked away from everything and said, 'Count me out.'

The WRC organisers said, 'What will you do?'

I said, 'I'm going back to Italy.'

They then said, 'You've played in Italy for a while, haven't you?'

'Yes.'

'Well, we'll give you the same amount of money to deliver the Italian team.'

My response was, 'Thank you very much; that's very flattering. But I'm a guest in that country and I don't want to be part of destroying rugby there either.'

I knew that the time had come for rugby to become professional and that this movement might prove to be the catalyst. I just didn't want to be a part of the process.

WITH ME OUT OF the picture, a few other senior players in Australia took over at the forefront of negotiations with WRC. Rumour has it there was pressure exerted on the younger Wallabies to sign. It's said they were brought into the WRC office individually and told something to the effect of, 'You've got to sign. We've got to be united, we're all in this together.' Whether or not that is true, in the end, thanks in part to the money being waved around, there were just three players, I believe, who'd been part of the World Cup squad who refused to sign the letters of intent: me, Tim Gavin and Jason Little.

Jason always liked to present himself as this naive, grass-chewing country boy from Toowoomba. He is a very bright fellow, always was, but he'd perfected the persona of someone who didn't quite know what was going on. He's a lovely guy and is now doing very well in his chosen field.

Everyone was battling over him in 1995. He said no to rugby league, said no to the rugby circus and instead became the poster boy for the Australian Rugby Union. They gave him a huge amount of money to become their first professional rugby signing. It was a smart move on Jason's part—he played each of the three parties off the other and got what he wanted. It was a no-lose situation for him, when you think about it. He was staying with the established body, getting paid and not jeopardising his international career.

As it turned out, the planned circus didn't happen anyway. All the other guys signed letters of intent with the WRC, but then it fell apart because in August 1995 rugby was declared an open (and professional) sport by the IRB. That put an end to the need for a breakaway. That's the short story.

At the same time—and I knew this was going on too—SANZAR (formed by the New Zealand, South African and Australian unions) signed a deal, under the name SANZAR initially; it would later become the Super 12 and then the Super 14 competitions. It was a US$550 million deal for ten years' worth of exclusive broadcasting rights. It was to start in 1996. It sounds like a lot of money, doesn't it? But at the time, I was thinking, 'Hmmm, I'm not sure how far that money will actually stretch.'

I remember sitting with Leo Williams, who was Chairman of the Australian Rugby Union. He has now, sadly, passed away.

He was saying, 'I've negotiated the biggest deal in Australian sporting history' and all that kind of thing.

I said, 'Leo, let's just look at the figures.'

It was US$550 million over ten years. That's US$55 million each year. Then you divide that by three countries. Within each of those three countries there were four teams that had to be sustained. When you look at it like that, it's not that much money. I'd say that News Corporation got an absolute bargain. But it saved rugby by preventing a big split, and saved a few players from going down the route of rugby league.

I'm sure I'm not generalising when I say that most rugby union players wouldn't particularly choose to go and play rugby league. They are two different games and two very different worlds. The main incentive to go to league was always money, but the professionalisation of rugby union levelled the playing field somewhat. I never had anything against league; I followed it and always caught up with a few guys I knew who played for the Queensland teams. Because it was so popular, you couldn't really avoid it. It was and is a much more popular code in Australia than rugby.

I even had a few offers from rugby league over the years. I remember one in particular. I can't remember the exact year; it was sometime in the late '80s.

I was sitting in my office in Brisbane one morning when the phone rang, pretty early—'Good morning, Michael Lynagh speaking.'

There was a lady on the other end with a pretty thick accent, clearly from somewhere in the north of England. She said, 'Is this the office of Michael Lynagh? Do you have a fax number?'

I said yes and gave it to her and she said that a Mr Joe Pickavance of St Helens rugby league club wanted to send a fax through to me. Of course I knew who he was because he was in the news a lot. St Helens were a big team at the time and a few Australians had gone over to play there.

So this piece of paper came through. For the time, it was a pretty amazing offer for a five-year contract. This guy had never even spoken to me, so it was obvious that this was merely an opening offer—something to test the water. I thought, 'Jeez, I need to think about this pretty seriously.' I can't remember how much it was, but for those days it was a lot of money, with more potentially waiting. I spoke to my father about it—'This could set me up for life.'

At the time I was captain of Queensland and vice-captain of Australia, doing well at work, and enjoying living in Brisbane, going surfing every weekend in the sun. Life was good. Dad said, 'Do you really want to give all that up to go and live in the north of England and get beaten up every week?' When he put it like that, the decision was easily made. And it didn't involve me signing for St Helens. Some things are more important than money, I realised. It's a belief I would stick to.

TWELVE

A CINDERELLA STORY

HAVING GONE BACK TO Italy for one last season after the 1995 World Cup, I was enjoying life without the pressures of international rugby. I yearned for very few aspects of it. I missed the guys, but certainly not the training or the tension before games. The frayed nerves. The feeling sick, worrying about whether the kicks would go over.

Instead of stressing about training, fitness, injuries and captaining a team, I was enjoying making plans with Isabella. We were engaged and planned to marry in July 1996. My arrangement at Treviso would soon be over, so we were pondering questions like, 'Where would we like to live?' It seemed as if, almost overnight, someone had removed my shackles. I was thirty-two years old and starting life all over again with a blank canvas. We were toying with the idea of moving back to Australia to live, but we had no firm plans. We were happy trying to map out where life might take us.

EVERY NIGHT AT TREVISO, the players would all go up to the rugby office before training in the evening. We'd have a coffee, have a chat and collect our mail. There was a letter from the UK waiting for me one night. As I rarely corresponded with anyone in the UK, I thought, 'This is unusual.'

It turned out to be from a guy who was involved with Saracens Rugby Club. The gist of his letter was, 'Would you be interested in coming to Saracens to play?' I'd never heard of Saracens, but I thought, 'Yeah, sounds interesting.'

So Isabella and I went over to meet Saracens' soon-to-be owner, Nigel Wray, in London in April. The letter confirming our travel arrangements said, 'You'll come over on the Friday, stay at this or that hotel and then there's two tickets for you to go and see *Riverdance*.'

I thought, 'What the hell is *Riverdance*?' and when I found out it was Irish folk dancing I wasn't at all excited—'God, that's the last thing I want to go and see.'

Of course, along we went and it was absolutely brilliant. We bought the CD, bought the program, bought the VHS—we loved it all. Then we met with Nigel on the Saturday over dinner at a nice restaurant in the West End called Quaglino's. It was a great night and I immediately liked Nigel and his wife, Linda, and felt I could trust him. Luckily, I think he felt the same way about me. On the Sunday we went to Nigel and Linda's house for lunch and continued to build our relationship.

Nigel grew up in North London and Saracens was his local club. I liked his vision for it. Not only did he want to create a great rugby club, he wanted to take it a step further and make it an all-encompassing sporting club with a wide range of facilities for members, like those in Argentina, for example. He was after an environment that transcended rugby. I completely bought into the idea and thought, 'I see where you're going with this. I want to be part of it.'

As we departed for the airport on the Sunday evening, the last thing Nigel said to me was: 'Here's my number. It would be great to have you on board. If there are any questions, just remember that the answer is always yes.'

I thought, 'That's a pretty nice thing for someone to say.'

Isabella and I went back to Italy to discuss things. Nigel had said, 'I see you being around for three to five years.' There was no contract at that stage. Nonetheless, both Isabella and I decided that we should commit to Saracens. We felt that London would be a nice but neutral place to start our married life together. I wouldn't be dragging her to Australia and she wouldn't be keeping me in Italy. London is a great city, and living there would be a challenge, but, as a couple, the decision really suited us.

NIGEL WRAY, OWNER OF SARACENS: When I got involved in Saracens, rugby was a pretty insular game. The same people were on the touchline and I didn't particularly want anybody else coming along. I thought we needed a signing that would create some interest. I also thought, mathematically, that someone like Michael Lynagh who scores 12 to 14 points a game would give us a good chance of not losing. We approached him and he joined us.

Isabella and I arrived in London after a honeymoon that took us to Australia, Hawaii and the mainland US. While we were in Brisbane, Isabella and I went and watched Australia playing New Zealand at Lang Park. It was less than a year since I'd retired.

Even then, with the smell of dressing rooms barely out of my system, I remember sitting in the stand and thinking, 'I'm so glad I'm up here watching this rather than being down in the dressing room, sitting with the guys, ready to run out.' It's moments like that when you know you've made the right decision in moving on. Not that I particularly needed confirmation; I'd been absolutely sure that the 1995 World Cup was the end for me, win or lose.

I remember arriving in London from New York at five in the morning at the end of our honeymoon. We'd already rented a flat in Hampstead, but it was unfurnished. So we'd gone out to Ikea and John Lewis and said, 'We'll be back on the 23rd of August and we need all this stuff to be delivered on that day.'

But before the deliveries arrived that morning, including basics like beds, wardrobes and cutlery, we sat on the floor of the flat, waiting for the local Tesco Metro supermarket to open so that we could buy some plastic bowls and some milk and cornflakes. We'd arrived with only our clothes and we built it up from there to where we are today. Our life in London is something we've created as a couple, and it has worked out very well for us.

I USED TO GET annoyed when I read about rugby mercenaries moving to England to play. They'd take the field for a year, not play very well, cash in and then go home. That was never part of the equation for me. The money was nice, sure, but it wasn't just about the rugby or the money. It was a lifestyle choice as much as a rugby decision. And it wasn't just my choice; it was Isabella's too. Not just that either: I really wanted to make a positive contribution to the Saracens' project and repay the trust that Nigel had placed in me.

Equally, it annoys me a little when I hear people say, 'It's not about the money. It's all about the culture and the experience.' Yeah, that's great—it is about experiencing new cultures and a new country. But money is important. If you're an engineer and you get asked to work in France or maybe Japan—of course it's about the money. It's a great opportunity as well, but if they weren't paying you anything, you wouldn't go, would you? It's all part of the melting pot you've got to throw everything into when you're making a decision about where you're going to live and work.

So for us, a move to London was about a whole series of things and I was fortunate enough to meet someone at the forefront of professional club rugby and to capitalise on that relationship. My relationship with Nigel Wray was and is a great thing and it changed my life. My life and Isabella's. And we're still living it.

I AGREED TO COME to Saracens on a handshake. Nigel and I could have got lawyers involved and contracts signed, but I said to him, 'I'm happy to trust you.' He said, 'That's good. I'm happy to trust you.' We shook hands on it and that was about it. Isabella and I upped sticks and moved to a new country. I always thought that it was a very strong start to a friendship and business relationship, and I think Nigel felt the same way.

NIGEL WRAY: It was very obvious to me immediately that Michael was a giver in life, not a taker. In those days, Saracens was very much a Cinderella side. There's no doubt that Michael could have joined what were perceived to be much better clubs. We were actually in danger of being relegated in that last season of amateur rugby in 1995 and I think he may have actually already been approached by other clubs around that time. But he had already agreed to come to us. When I asked him, he said, 'Even if Saracens do get relegated, I still stick to my word. I'm coming to play for you.' That's the type of man Michael Lynagh is.

A couple of months later we had an exchange of letters. He sent me one—it was no more than two pages long. I signed it, kept a copy and sent him the original back. That was it. Nigel Wray kept all his promises over all the time I was at Saracens and to this day he continues to be very generous. I'd like to think that I did the same.

I started playing in September 1996. I was in pretty good physical shape. I'd taken my training gear on honeymoon and we'd stayed at nice places where it was pleasant to run. I had a house at Sunshine Beach, near Noosa in Queensland, so we'd stayed there for the initial part of the honeymoon—running along the beach, surfing. Then we did the same thing in Hawaii.

When we arrived in Los Angeles, we hired a car and drove up the Pacific Coast Highway to San Francisco. It's one of the best drives in the world—from Malibu up through Big Sur. I couldn't take my eyes off the ocean.

Along the way we stopped in the Monterey peninsula for a couple of days. It's a seventeen-mile stretch of amazingly rugged coastline. It's just beautiful; I'd happily live there. I got up every day feeling energised and went running around Cypress Point, Pebble Beach and Spyglass Hill—fabulous golf courses that I'd only ever seen on TV. I'd say to Isabella, 'I'm going for a run.'

But the real purpose was to see these great golf courses—'I'll kill two birds with one stone here ...'

So by the time I arrived at Saracens for the first season, sometime in mid-August, I was in a more than decent state of physical fitness. Not match-fit by any stretch of the imagination, but a few pre-season training sessions would soon see to that, I thought. The first official training session at Southgate Park was memorable for a couple of reasons. It's a public oval in North London with just a small stand and clubhouse, and I remember we all had to wander around the pitch picking up dog shit before we started. I'd never done that before and there was quite a lot of it. I remember thinking, 'So this is professional rugby?' Other than the mess on the pitch, it was really no different from what I was accustomed to.

People have told me that George Chuter—who would later play a few games for England—tells a good story on the after-dinner circuit about that first session. He was there as a fresh-faced youngster. He was just nineteen and this was his first-ever training session with a professional club. He was there on trial, I think. Apparently I walked into the Saracens dressing room for my first training session and George is sitting there in a replica Australia jersey. He says that I just looked him up and down and said, 'Nice jersey, mate', before jogging out to the training ground. He was probably thinking, 'Here's Michael Lynagh, however many international caps, and there I am in an Australia jersey. A replica jersey at that!'

There was a strange atmosphere for the first few sessions. It felt like some kind of boarding-school initiation was being played out and that I was being scrutinised. I think some of the old guard were a little suspicious of guys like me, Philippe

Sella, Kyran Bracken and all the other high-profile new recruits turning up. I'm sure some of them thought, 'So what if he's got seventy-two caps; let's see what he's really made of.'

The thing is, I'd already addressed that issue in my mind. I'd assessed how I might be perceived and had thought about how I'd respond. The last thing I wanted anyone to think was that I was there to wind my career down and collect a nice fat pay cheque for good measure. That idea never even entered my head. I was there to do a job for the period I'd agreed and that, to me, meant total commitment to the task. If anything, I was determined to over-achieve. I did much more than necessary in the way of training, more in the way of preparation, so that there could be no doubt in anyone's mind as to my motives.

George's story also talks about the tackling drill we did at that first training session. Cones were put out to make a square, roughly 25 metres by 25 metres. Half of the thirty guys who were there that night lined up in one corner; the other half in the opposite corner. One group was attacking; the other was to defend. As the guys went through their paces, some tried tricky moves to beat their defender, whereas others kept it simple, with strong, direct running. When my turn to defend came round, Charlie Olney was standing in the opposite corner. As he got ready—scraping his foot on the ground, almost like a bull—I could sense a few of the old guard looking at each other as if to say, 'Here we go, boys.' I've often wondered if it was staged—'Let's get a 100-kilo-plus hooker to run at the highly paid prima donna.'

What these guys didn't know, but soon would, was that I was no prima donna. I didn't particularly fancy Olney's fast-moving, 100-kilo bulk running at me, but refusal, or indeed any adverse reaction, just wasn't an option. There was a lot riding on my actions.

So I grabbed him around the legs as he approached and put him to the floor with a textbook tackle. No dump-tackling, no drama—just a correctly executed tackle. Then I calmly jogged back to my corner, showing no signs of effort. I just did what was required. And from that moment on, I had the total respect of everyone. All their doubts were removed. My commitment or motives were never questioned thereafter. After that, I'm sure they were thinking, 'Okay, this Lynagh's the real deal.'

It was a very significant moment, but it probably wouldn't happen nowadays, because the arrangement of bringing internationals into club sides is completely understood. Nobody is going to stand Dan Carter in a square and ask Bismarck du Plessis to run at him. The game has moved on from those old-fashioned rites of initiation.

That said, I admit that I'm not a physical person; I don't like being hurt. Who does? Yet I played rugby for fifteen years. Getting hit went hand in hand with it. But physical contact was an aspect of playing rugby that I never really relished. I actually got really nervous about it in the days before a game. I worried about it during the game too. I was never particularly big and there were always, all the way through my career, people running at me—trying to get to me. I got round it by thinking, 'Right, I know I'm going to be run at by big people. I'm going to get hit. Targeted.' You've just got to close your eyes and do your best. What I never wanted was a reputation as a guy who shirks tackles—a turnstile letting everyone through. Once you got that reputation, you were in trouble: you'd be targeted even more as a potential weak link.

They'd just run at you all day—'Let's run over the top of this guy.'

Jonny Wilkinson, a modern great player in my position, took it to the other extreme for a while. He seemed to relish clobbering people, often injuring himself in the process. A few flyhalves nowadays have followed his lead. The position is much more confrontational than it used to be, and Wilkinson's a big reason why. It almost looked as if he viewed defence as a personal challenge—'Run at me if you dare.' People took him on and got hammered. Thereafter it was, 'Well, I'm not running down his channel anymore.'

I always thought, 'All right mate, we know you can tackle. You can slow down now. You're of more value to the team when you're on the field, not sitting in the stand, injured.' But that was just the way he was. I wasn't like that by nature. Alan Jones, our Wallaby coach up until 1988, said to me once, when he saw me getting too physically involved in a game: 'You're a thoroughbred; you don't belong in there.' Anytime I got stressed about tackling in a game, I just thought about my friends up there in the forwards. The Tommy Lawtons, Phil Kearnses and David Wilsons of the world. Now when *they* tackle you, that's a physical confrontation. I used to say to myself, 'You think you have it hard. Imagine how they are feeling.' That's how I got through it. The actual running of the game and making decisions never worried me a bit. If that had been all I had to do, I'd probably still be doing it now.

The few occasions that I played centre, mostly playing outside Mark Ella in the early 1980s, actually helped my defence a little. All of a sudden I had to make tackles against bigger men than me, whereas a flyhalf in those days was mostly cover defending, picking up chip kicks, that kind of thing. All of that suited me fine. I used to say that defence for a flyhalf in those days was more managerial than physical. And I was very good at managing other people to make tackles for me. I never shirked, but making hits just wasn't my forte.

In retrospect, I don't blame the Sarries guys for wanting to test me physically. It was the very early days of professional rugby and nobody really knew how bringing in highly paid players from overseas would work out. I would have tested me too!

NIGEL WRAY: I'd only seen Michael play on the great stages. We all had. But somehow it was even more impressive to see him play up close on a small pitch at Enfield. His hands were just incredible to watch. I thought that the first time he trained. If you watched his hands, you just never knew whether he was going to give a short pass or a long pass. He also had incredible awareness of where to put a rugby ball. He had that in spades.

But the key to that first season at Saracens wasn't simply that they brought in big names. It was much more to do with exactly which big names they acquired—the right kinds of personalities, not just good rugby players. Anyone can go out and acquire big names. Lots of teams did it. Some worked out, some were disasters—and the ones that didn't work were usually because the players concerned were there with the wrong agenda.

ROB ANDREW: This is where everything moved so quickly. You went from a World Cup in South Africa to almost signing up for a rugby circus. Then the IRB said the game was professional, almost overnight. Everybody just looked at each other and went,

'Blimey, now what?' In England, people stepped in and bought clubs: Newcastle United via Sir John Hall bought the old Gosforth Rugby club, which then became Newcastle Falcons. Things moved at a frightening pace. I was working as a chartered surveyor in London. I got a call on a Wednesday asking if I wanted to come to Newcastle, and by the following Monday I'd decided to go. The financial incentive was there, but there was also a game-changing decision to be made about what I was going to do next. When I look back on it now, it was a bit like the Wild West for the first few years. Nobody knew how it was going to play out. Everyone just jumped on the bandwagon, but nobody really knew where it was going. Michael and I were in right at the beginning, right at the end of our careers. 1995 will go down in history as the key year in the game. We just happened to straddle that period.

By approaching guys like myself, Philippe Sella and, later that year, Francois Pienaar, Nigel Wray had chosen extremely wisely in his first year of running a professional rugby team. It was a combination of good judgement and a big slice of luck. While all three of us are completely different types of people, we all went to Saracens with the view that we were there to do a job. We weren't there just for the money; we were there to train hard, play hard on the weekend and do the very best for the team. We all wanted to leave a footprint by being part of something exciting.

Even the ever-laidback Philippe, whom you wouldn't necessarily see as someone who'd relish training in the freezing cold on a Monday night on a dog-shit minefield in North London, was there to do well. He's an easygoing kind of guy, yes. But he also knew his job and took it very seriously.

It didn't matter that he was approaching the end of his brilliant career. He trained and played as if he was on trial, like George Chuter. He had language issues to deal with, something I knew all about from my time in Italy, but he fitted in like anyone else. He was one of the boys—just a really popular guy.

I remember one week we played up in Rotherham. We gave all the backs' moves a name, and we decided to call one of them that we used a lot 'Rotherham'. Well, Philippe couldn't for the life of him say the word 'Rotherham'. I think we called it that to wind him up a little. I'd say 'Rotherham!' and then Philippe would have to pass the information on to the wingers outside him. His English was fine, but Rotherham isn't exactly the easiest word to say if you're French—'Rrrrrrr ...' In fairness to him, I'm sure there are plenty of English-speaking people who can't say it.

On the field, Philippe was very special. Sometimes you'd put him in a position where you'd bring a fullback in and have Philippe drifting wide. You'd pass the ball all the way across to Philippe and all he needed was the defender to have a quick look at the fullback inside—and he was gone. We had to adapt our way of playing because he just wasn't used to structure. Being a bit-part player within an intricate move wasn't something he was accustomed to. We had those moves, but most of them ended up with Philippe getting the ball at the end of them anyway. He was a very important player.

Despite the shrewd personnel signings, the first year at Saracens wasn't a total success. The team didn't go as well as it probably could have, and for the first time in my career I got some niggling injuries that just wouldn't clear up. Besides, we were all just dipping our toes into professionalism, testing the waters. A lot of guys were still working and then we were training at night, out at Southgate. I, too, was working in that early period. I'd said to Nigel at one of our meetings, 'By the way, I've always worked when I've been playing.' He said, 'Really? What do you do?' I said, 'Property.' And he said, 'I'm chairman of a commercial property investment company here called Burford.'

So Nigel introduced me to a lovely fellow called Nick Leslau, who ran Burford—he was the CEO. I started working for the company in October 1996, in their Marylebone office. But I soon found that working in the West End and then trying to get out to Southgate to train in the evening was causing both work and rugby to suffer. So I went to Nick and Nigel and said, 'Look, I can't do both. The travelling is killing me. We're professionals and there's a lot of young guys out there who I'm struggling to keep up with as it is. I'm not as fit as I could be and I'm tired. I'm here to play rugby, so let me concentrate on that and we'll come back to business later.'

They completely respected my decision, not to mention my honesty. It was true. I *was* there to play rugby. I was also thirty-three. It was a wise and sensible move for all of us. In order to do myself justice and keep up with guys who were ten years younger than me, I had to focus one hundred per cent on getting myself in the best shape I could be in.

Despite being one of the older guys, I liked everyone in the Saracens squad. It was a very good mixture of youth and experience. However, for the first time in my career, I actually *felt* older. It wasn't as if suddenly I thought I couldn't compete. It was subtler than that—more an acknowledgement of the fact that my priorities had changed a little bit. It shouldn't have come as a great surprise given what I'd been through in the last year and a half.

There were guys at Saracens who were nineteen, twenty, twenty-one—thrusting, wide-eyed and keen to the possibilities. I was too, but I was thirty-three, with a lot of miles on the clock and a new wife at home. There was a difference. So to go nightclubbing in central London every weekend wasn't high on my agenda. But I certainly didn't begrudge any of the guys who wanted to do that. If I'd been in their position, with a bit of money, as they now had, I'd have been in there with them as well. But my social needs had changed. I wanted something else from life. I had a wife, a home; I was keen to nurture that because I knew that it was my future after rugby.

Amazingly, it was at Saracens that for the first time in my rugby career I was subjected to a curfew. During all the tours I'd been on with Australia or Queensland, nobody had ever told us when to go to bed. It still blows my mind thinking about it.

We were up in Newcastle and then Scotland for some pre-season training and games, staying in a hotel. As we were standing in the foyer one evening, about to go out, our manager said, 'Right, everyone, back by midnight.' I looked at Philippe as if to say, 'Did I hear that correctly?' and Philippe said, 'What? I don't even finish dinner by midnight.'

We came back at around eleven-thirty and the Saracens management were sitting in the foyer of the hotel, ticking players off a list as they returned. I felt like a twelve-year-old at St Joseph's all over again. I also felt that it was the wrong thing to do, for a couple of reasons. First, people resented it and it created a bit of an 'us and them' environment—

like teachers and pupils, where we, the players, weren't considered by management to be adult enough to make our own decisions.

Secondly, if you've got some guy who goes out until four in the morning when he's meant to be training at nine, you soon work out whether he's the guy you want in your team. If he can't be responsible for his actions in the pre-season, then maybe he's not the guy for you. I'd actually rather find out that way. But instead, asking everyone to be back by twelve and then giving someone who gets back at half past twelve extra laps to do ... I think that defeats the purpose.

I've thought about it since, and while I originally considered the curfew to be a product of the professional game, I now think it was more of a control thing, unique at that time to the UK—'We'd better keep some kind of control on these blokes or else we'll lose them—they'll *never* come home.'

By the way, I would agree with that in the case of some of the younger guys—they might indeed have never come back. But at least you'd soon know. I just thought to myself, 'I'd rather watch and see who *doesn't* come home.' In that situation, you would have probably found that some of the young guys stayed out a bit late. But then the next day they'd do extra; put in more work or whatever was needed to make amends. I'm all for some give and take among adults.

But if you've got someone who's come in at five, stumbling around and can't play—'Aw coach, my hamstring's a bit tight'— you're not going to pick him in a big game, are you? Going out and having a good time is absolutely fine, I've always thought that. But, like anything, there's always a time and a place—like after the game on a Saturday.

I thought the curfew was part of the same culture as the tackling drill. It was a way of making sure that everyone was treated the same—particularly guys like me and Philippe. Fortunately, I also recognised, in both cases, that if I didn't keep quiet and do as I was told, my season wouldn't be much fun. But I'm sure there were plenty of foreign players around at that time who wouldn't have responded like that. They'd have thought, 'Tackling drill? I don't have to do that. Curfew? I'm not obeying that.' That would only have led to resentment and a lack of unity on the pitch.

I knew that I had to be the opposite of the typical 'star', and for me it wasn't difficult. I felt that I had approached the latter years of my international career as if I was already professional. I'd managed my life in a way that might be expected of a professional in any field. I was organised, courteous, considerate and honest. Part of it was my upbringing; another part was a result of the various decisions I'd made in my life and the rewards I'd got for making them. I had a great marriage, and healthy relationships with my clubs, unions and my fellow players. I never in my life went into a situation thinking, 'What can I get out of this?' Instead I always thought, 'This is great. This has worked. What can we do *next* year?'

In fact, I don't go into relationships of any kind thinking about when they will end. I'm always thinking about how they can be nurtured, developed and sustained. There's a big difference and not a lot of people do it.

TIM HORAN: We always used to admire Noddy for how he created great relationships all over the world. The values he had and the friendships he created off the field were as important as his playing ability. He had a huge role in my development regarding how you handle yourself with the Wallaby jersey on, but also when you finish playing. There's still an ambassadorial role to play and Noddy was the role model.

FRANCOIS PIENAAR ARRIVED AT Saracens in December 1996. He was another shrewd acquisition, a guy who came with every intention of doing his absolute best for the team, with no desire to hitch a free ride. Francois was a big character. He was a World Cup-winning captain and the kind of guy who, whenever he gets involved in something, takes it on, takes total control of it and does it to a very high standard. He does that in every aspect of his life.

Francois played for the 1996–97 season and later became player–coach, taking over from Mark Evans. Francois' approach was very different from Mark's, and a lot of people didn't initially like it. I personally liked him and I got his approach. He was very confident and dominant in his style and very much a winner in terms of his views on discipline and training. He'd just won a World Cup and his team were definitely the fittest group in the competition. Who could argue with that?

That second pre-season in 1997, I trained as hard as I ever remember training in my life. It was a really tough regime. We were running a lot, carrying bricks around, jumping—we were unbelievably fit. I was very fit too, with no sign of the niggling injuries of the year before. That's how Francois had won the 1995 World Cup: the South Africans were by far the fittest team there. He brought all those methods with him, and he was a very inspirational speaker as well.

Some players didn't particularly like his enthusiastic coaching style, or him, and that meant that I gradually became a buffer between Francois and some members of the squad. Sometimes when Francois was pushing too hard, I'd go to him and say, 'Look, the guys are tired', 'The guys don't like this or that', 'That's not going to go down well.' Equally, I might say, 'He needs his arse kicked' or 'Mate, it's time to put the foot down.' He was getting a lot of feedback from me that he trusted and the players knew that too. It worked pretty well.

The upshot of the training regime was that the results were much better in my second season. People can complain about training regimes all day if they like, but if the results are good and the style of rugby is attractive, it's hard for anyone to argue too much with the methods. Guys who were whining in August about having to do ten consecutive fireman lifts would be saying in January, 'You know what, this is all right.' Nobody likes change, but once the players started seeing results from an individual point of view and a team point of view, they accepted it a lot more readily.

On a personal level, I was developing my 'I'll prepare in the best way I can for every game' mode. There were plenty of cold and wet days when I would have much rather been doing other things, and when the other guys were sitting inside, but I'd get out there, practising my goal-kicking. No discussion, no fanfare; just good, structured preparation. And it paid off. I was kicking better than I ever had and because of it the team's results were better. It wasn't all down to me, as it never should be, but by kicking at 80 per cent plus that season I was more than pulling my weight. It *felt* better too. I'm not saying the pressure was gone, but there's definitely something to be said for turning up at a game knowing that you've done everything you possibly could have in advance. I still kicked on feel, but the difference was that there was a bit more planning to back it up.

AS GOOD AS THINGS were at Saracens during that 1997 season, I realised around January or February 1998 that it was going to be my last season playing rugby. I was playing well, enjoying myself and holding together physically, but the thought of another pre-season made me decide to retire. I'd reached a point, quite reasonably I think, where I was having to work too hard to keep up with the younger guys, and I didn't think I had the stomach for going through it all again.

A month before the season ended, I had conversations with Nigel Wray and Nick Leslau and we agreed that once I'd finished at Saracens I'd go straight back into working in commercial property at Prestbury, a company Nick and Nigel had recently started. I liked that feeling of having something new to go to. It was the next chapter in my life and I was really looking forward to it.

Even before it happened, it felt right. Just as in 1995, I knew it was the right decision. Fortunately, having gone close to winning the premiership in 1997, but narrowly coming second to Rob Andrew's Newcastle Falcons, Philippe (who'd also decided to retire) and I would get the opportunity to sign off on the best possible stage: the Tetley Bitter Cup final against Wasps.

There was a huge build-up to that Cup final at Twickenham. Win, lose or draw, it was going to be the last time I ever played competitive rugby and there was a lot of pressure and press attention because of that. It was a big deal for Saracens too, because it was the first Cup final they'd ever appeared in. Everything pointed to it being a fabulous occasion: my last game, Philippe's last game and the Cinderella team of English rugby in the final of the Cup. I thought, 'Okay, mate, this is it.'

We ended up staying in the same hotel out in Weybridge as the Wallabies had in 1991, before the World Cup final. When we arrived there, I looked around and thought, 'I think I've been here before.' It was a little different after seven years; there'd been some building development in the area immediately around the hotel. But on the morning of the match, I decided to go for a walk, to see if I could find that same hill where I'd kicked balls back in '91. I found it, and did exactly the same thing again.

I remember walking down the tunnel for the final quite vividly. My stomach was in knots as I walked out, but literally the moment that the sunlight hit my face as I walked onto the pitch and saw the huge crowd I smiled and said to myself, 'Welcome home. You're in your office. You know what you're doing—off you go.' It was really liberating.

If that's the way you feel, you know that you should retire. I played really well, physically I was okay and we won the game 48–18. It couldn't have worked out better.

Journalists afterwards said, 'You played great! Are you going to play next year now? ' I said, 'No, it's *because* I played great that I'm not playing again.' That's the way I wanted to be remembered. Also, and every bit as importantly, that was how I wanted to remember myself. That was exactly how I wanted to go out, feeling calm and thinking, 'This is my stage.' Not just that, I felt I had achieved what Nigel brought me to Saracens to do. He wanted to put this little North London club on the map—and by beating Wasps in a final at Twickenham we had certainly done that.

I've talked to Nigel often about Saracens since I left. As an outsider, it's easy to observe what's really going on. After Philippe and I left, things didn't quite reach the heights of that 1997–98 season for a long time. I think Nigel believed that the secret of success was simply to go out and buy big-name players with a hundred caps. I've said to him on more than one occasion, 'The biggest problem you had is that it did work in the first year and you thought that was the formula.' He sees that now, but it took him a while, with a few wrong choices along the way.

In fact Saracens bought in players for ten years after I left, and it didn't work every time. The reason? They didn't always bring in the right personalities.

Some people came in to the club and did the bare minimum and collected the money. They thought, 'Let's see what I can get away with here.' They wouldn't give a hundred per cent because they didn't want to get injured; that would have influenced their salary. That's the wrong attitude to bring to a club. I've often wondered whether that attitude was a product of the professional game. Once players became more used to professional life, maybe some of them thought, 'Let's just go through the motions and take the money.'

Nowadays I see Saracens as being much closer to the vision Nigel had at the start. People refer to 'the cult of Saracens' and while I think that's a bit strong, I do see a clear club ethos that you either buy into or you leave. It's very much focused on working together, doing everything together and being very inclusive of family. The argument is—and I believe in it—that if players are happy in every aspect of their lives, they'll play better. It's a close-knit group; they're all in it together. The theory being that when it gets really tough on the weekend, you're more inclined to play for the guys beside you. That's the kind of ethos they've developed over the last four or five years. Players are coming there not to see what they can get out of it. They're there to *give* something back and to make Saracens a better place than it was when they arrived. That's a very hard ethos to establish in a professional club.

When I look at Toulon, it always surprises me that they've managed to create a similar ethos in a club that brings in superstars. But when I give it more thought, I can't help believing that Jonny Wilkinson is a big part of the reason they've managed it. In many ways, the way he approached his time at Toulon was very similar to how I operated at Saracens—only Jonny went on and applied a whole new level of dedication.

At Toulon you've got guys who've got a hundred caps and are reaching the end of their careers. They're in the south of France, thinking, 'This is nice.' They're getting paid good money for being there, too, yet there's Jonny out training and practising for six hours every single day. Watching him, they must think, 'Oh, this really *means* something to him', and so they've started doing the same thing.

It has all evolved very quickly and I don't think it was any surprise that the two clubs that ended up in the final of the 2014 Heineken Cup were Saracens and Toulon. They've both got pretty good players, yes, but they've also got the strongest ethos and culture. Having met a lot of the current Saracens guys, I know that ethos and culture is a very big part of their make-up. The club feels like a family.

It always irritates me when journalists make blanket statements about professional rugby. Recently a guy at *The Telegraph* published something that included me among players who'd come to England just to make money. I had an illuminating exchange with him, and it's very rare that I feel the need to do that. I felt my integrity, values and honesty were being called into question, so I phoned him and said, 'Mate, I still live here, for a start.' Then I said, 'And go and ask any one of my teammates how hard I worked.' Finally I said, 'You're absolutely right about what you say. Some people *did* come with that attitude. But don't put my name in among them.'

Did he apologise? No. He said, 'Point taken. I didn't really mean it like that. But you were a big name …' I said, 'A big name maybe, but I've still got a reputation that means something to me. So don't bracket me where I don't deserve to be.'

We left it at that.

THIRTEEN

BLINDSIDED

I CONTINUED TO WORK in England with Nick Leslau for Prestbury Investment Holdings and began working for Sky, commenting on Premiership games on the weekends, in 1998. In 2000, we moved back to Italy so that Isabella could be close to family and friends. I'd travel back and forth to work for both Sky and Prestbury, according to how my meeting schedule looked. It worked really well for a couple of years, and whenever I came over for any length of time—three weeks or more—Isabella and our son, Louis, would come with me and we'd stay in the two-bedroom flat in Mayfair that I bought in 2001. It was a great little place, with car parking right in the centre of London. I got it for a really good price.

I remember flying home from Australia on the morning of 9/11. I was in Paris, going through to Venice. In line with me were a whole group of passengers who were waiting to connect to New York. I was lucky. I got on my flight, landed in Venice, went home and fell asleep on the couch.

Sometime in the afternoon, Isabella woke me up, saying, 'Look at this, look at this!' Dazed and jetlagged, I opened my eyes. It was just around the time that the second plane was hitting. I said, 'What did you wake me up to watch a *Die Hard* movie for?' And she said, 'No, it's real!' That was it, I sat watching for the whole day as the events unfolded.

I had to travel to London the next day. Originally Isabella and Louis were going to come with me, but I ended up going on my own. I've never seen a flight so empty. There was almost no traffic on the road on the drive from Heathrow either; it was a very eerie atmosphere. Our flat was very close to the US Embassy. I remember getting up very early one morning, jetlagged, and wandering over to Grosvenor Square. There was a book of condolences there for the public to sign; I remember feeling extremely emotional about it all. All those innocent people in the financial district who lost their lives, and those who died on the planes. I thought about the people in the queue in Paris heading for New York too. They probably would have been stuck there while US airspace went into lockdown. It's situations like that that make you thankful you weren't in the wrong place at the wrong time.

The commuting continued for another couple of years. It was tiring, but it was a good way of getting the best of both worlds. I could do my Sky work on the weekend and schedule some meetings on the Monday or Tuesday, then zip back to Italy on the early-morning flight from Gatwick and be sitting at home by mid-morning. It worked really well.

Then Thomas arrived in 2003 and it became more problematic for Isabella to travel with two young kids. Also, I got a bit worn down by it and found that, more and more, the opportunities in the UK were better than sitting in Italy, as nice a place as it is. Also, Louis was getting to the age where he was saying, 'Daddy's going away again?' It just wasn't fair on anybody. So Isabella and I discussed it and we both said, 'Why don't we go back to living in London?'

We'd sold the flat in Mayfair. It went very quickly. It had gone up in value massively and we couldn't justify sitting on it. I thought it would be much better to cash in and have the money in the bank. I guess I looked at what that flat was worth in comparison to what you'd get for the equivalent money in Australia and thought, 'This is crazy!' I still miss that flat, though. We had a lot of happy times there and I wish that I still owned it. Instead, we stayed in hotels in London until we decided to move back permanently.

We'd enjoyed living in Hampstead when I'd first arrived to play for Saracens but we also had some friends who lived in Richmond. The Sky studios were close by at that time too, and it seemed a great place to bring up a family. It's a lovely area, so in the summer of 2004 I took Isabella there for a weekend to have a look at a few houses.

We had a Pimm's on Richmond Green, sitting outside a beautiful old pub called The Cricketers. It was a glorious summer evening; there was cricket being played on the green … We said to each other, 'It's not a bad place, is it?'

Then we went for a walk along the river, had a nice dinner somewhere and it was at that point that we said, 'Richmond's all right. I think we could live here!' We bought a house, had some work done on it and then moved from Italy in July 2005. We've been in the London area ever since. I continued working with Nick and Nigel at Prestbury until 2006, when our youngest son, Nicolo, was born. Then I got an offer from my good friend David Coe (who passed away, sadly, in 2013) to take up a position with an Australian firm called the Allco Finance Group. I worked with Allco for the next couple of years. David and I had met while I was working with Robert Jones Investments back in 1990—we'd had a close friendship ever since and he was best man at my wedding.

WHEN THE FINANCIAL MARKET crashed in 2008, the Allco Finance Group went under, triggering the closure of the London office where I was working. For me it had been a full-time, five days a week job: assisting with setting up a European property fund, attempting to raise capital, searching for deals—the whole gamut of commercial property work. I was reasonably senior; it was a big commitment and, in addition, I was working for Sky on the weekends. For a guy with a young family you could say my plate was very full.

And then, in the summer of 2008, the black clouds appeared on the horizon of the entire financial market. Because we were the UK office of an Australian parent company, we were a little distant from the issues. We weren't kept in the dark; we just weren't facing bleak news head-on every day as they were in Sydney. In a sense that wasn't such a bad thing. In Australia, Allco was on the front page of every newspaper. In London, if I was at a dinner party and I told people where I worked, they probably wouldn't have even heard of Allco.

Morale was low, though, and I recall taking the London office for a night out to cheer the staff up and to talk to them about their fears—I just wanted to support them. The uncertainty was really starting to unsettle the Allco workers, and it wasn't just us—the whole world was in the same state of fear. Then, when Lehmans went under in September 2008, everything started to collapse. That was the tipping point of the whole process. It was a huge moment. All the staff in the London office of Allco, including me, lost their jobs. I felt terrible for everyone.

For the first few months of 2009, with the entire financial market having fallen off the edge of a cliff, I have to admit that things were pretty scary for us as a family. I'd lost my main source of income and was trying to get a new job by going round all my contacts in the commercial property world, and other sectors. I had a lot of those. While everyone was very helpful, they were all pretty nervous about their own jobs and if they were doing anything, they were cutting staff at that time, not looking to hire. There were just no jobs around and for the first time that I can remember, I had no real idea what to do next.

On reflection, that period taught me an awful lot about how people behave when put under extreme pressure. To see normally calm people climbing over others to save themselves was quite the eye-opener. It's not something I'd ever want to go through again, but the lessons I learned were very useful and clear. It seemed to me that when the pressure was on the concept of teamwork went out the window for some people. Understandably I suppose, a few people retreated into themselves and started looking out only for their futures. It was interesting to see who did what under pressure. The scenario reminded me of the 1995 World Cup quarter-final against South Africa. Everyone deals with stressful situations differently and I logged that information for future reference.

People say, 'When one door closes, another one opens', but that's not always the case in the economic market. One door shuts, they all shut. I wouldn't say I got down about losing my job and not quickly being able to find another, but I did ask myself a few questions. Most importantly: 'How can I turn this around?'

In one of quite a few periods of deep reflection and self-evaluation—the kind of staring-unblinkingly-into-the-fire mood you end up in when you lose your job and have a young family to support—I came to the realisation that the one currency I would always have is who I am. That's not meant to sound in any way arrogant or egotistical; it's just a fact of life. People know who I am. So, combining that fact with my decent background in business, I thought to myself: 'How can I use these strengths to my advantage in a business sense?'

The obvious solution was to take on the sort of role commonly taken up by ex-sportsmen, whereby my name, network and reputation would be used by a company to make introductions and forge relationships with others.

To be honest, it was the kind of role I'd intentionally steered away from in the past. I didn't want to be sixty years of age and still relying on something I did back in 1984 to make my living. In the same way, I have absolutely no problem with the after-dinner circuit and I'm very happy to have it as an option, but I didn't want it to be my living. That's just a personal choice. Lots of guys do choose that as a way of earning money after their playing careers end and most of them are very good at it and like doing it. I've been in the audience at a few of these dinners and I always enjoy them. But it wasn't what I wanted to do. I wanted to achieve something else. The ex-player side of things would always be in the background as a nice bonus if I needed it.

I felt the same way about going back to play rugby in a social capacity. Even now, when I'm down at Richmond on a Sunday with the kids, a lot of the dads and coaches from the boys' school play for the Richmond Heavies. They're always going, 'Why don't you come down and play?' My knees are so bad nowadays that I can hardly run, but on top of that I have absolutely no desire. I think that rugby for older guys is a great thing and should be encouraged, but it's not something I've ever been interested in doing. I always felt that I'd had my fill of getting knocked around on the field. Also, I've always had a feeling that there's bound to be one guy in any opposing team who'll think, 'Here's Michael Lynagh. Let's give him a bit of a hit.' Then he'd tell all his mates about it in the pub later.

I think that the key for me is that I've always kept rugby in its place. It's given me a huge amount, but I've never felt that it should define me as a person. It's something that I did, not who I am.

I was at a lunch the other day and I met this guy who said he'd met Lawrence Dallaglio, the former England captain, at a function, but hadn't previously known who he was. This guy openly admitted to Lawrence that he knew nothing about him. My first thought was, 'I bet that was really refreshing for Lawrence.'

I attend a lot of functions and when I sit down beside someone and they say, 'Look, I know nothing about rugby', I go, 'Ah, thank God! How nice.' Any slight pressure there might have been is suddenly off me—'Let's talk about something else. That would be really good.' Amusingly, some people I meet actually *apologise* for not having any knowledge of or interest in rugby. There's no need—I always love to talk about other subjects.

I'm not saying that it's bad to talk about rugby or that I'm not happy to. I'll admit that I used to wish I could resist conversations about it, but then I realised that I couldn't run from my rugby career. It will always be part of me and in some cases it's actually a very useful common ground when I first meet someone in a business situation. I'll talk about it and enjoy doing it. But I have plenty of interests outside it too.

I've never had a desire to coach, either. I like helping people, but not necessarily in a formal, structured capacity. You see a lot of the guys go back and coach goal-kicking—that's great. Passing on knowledge is always good. I've done a bit of it. But I think I'd find it a little frustrating, being a guy for whom things came reasonably easy from a natural ability perspective. Also, I'd rather not be tied to a week-in-week-out coaching situation when I had other things I wanted to do.

From a rugby perspective, the Sky stuff was keeping me involved at precisely the level I wanted. I like the game; I like watching the game. My Sky work wasn't a seven days a week thing, but at the same time it maintained my profile, not just in rugby, but in all aspects of business and personal life. Just to walk away from rugby and never have anything to do with it again would have been difficult, and a little unrealistic. To keep it going on the media side was as much as I wanted.

So what else *did* I want?

Well, I'd always wanted to create what I considered to be a 'new' Michael Lynagh—Michael Lynagh the property person who used to play a bit of rugby, as opposed to all the emphasis being on my rugby identity.

But given the situation I was in, I didn't have too many options. I wasn't going to sit around waiting for things to happen. I'm not good at that. I always like to have some kind of plan in place so I decided that I had to use what I had at my disposal: the currency of *me*. I should say, too, that I was very lucky to have the Sky TV work in the background, because it at least kept some cash coming in. My former colleagues in the commercial property and finance sector weren't as lucky. They were unemployed with few prospects, and I really felt for them.

So, over the year and a half or so after Allco collapsed, I created a portfolio of companies that were happy to use me as a means of being introduced to other companies. In some cases I sat on the board as a non-executive member, because I thought that the more involved I was, the better chance I had of getting traction when forming business relationships.

I feel it's much better to be able to say: 'Look, my name is Michael Lynagh and I'm a non-executive director on the board of this or that company …' than calling a business person and saying, 'Hi, I'm doing some work for company X …' or worse, 'I met Joe Bloggs at Tesco the other day. He makes widgets and you are a buyer of widgets. Let's all get together …' I personally feel that it gives you far more credibility as well as an enhanced knowledge of the company generally, and I always tried to promote that. I was hopeful that my idea would open a few doors for me, but I also knew that I'd probably need to be more proactive than I'd ever been before. Preparation was the key.

I had to research and understand the minutiae of not only the companies I was approaching, but also the particular individuals within those companies who made the key decisions. With the whole global economy shaken up by the economic downturn, it became obvious to me that my proven organisational, leadership and teamwork skills—on the rugby pitch as well as in subsequent roles—were the qualities that might open a few doors for me. I was determined to make these attributes that I'd spent a lifetime developing work in my favour.

AS PART OF THIS reinvention process, I had to do a fair bit of travelling, though I wasn't exactly thrilled at the prospect of spending more time away from Isabella and the kids. Our youngest son, Nicolo, was six and Louis and Thomas were getting to the age when they increasingly needed their dad around. I knew that and I felt the tug of regret every time I went away, but these were tough times and I had my family's financial wellbeing to consider. Like it or not, I *had* to put myself out there to network and one such trip involved a few meetings and opportunities in Singapore.

So on Tuesday 10th April 2012 I was on my way to Singapore for a speaking and networking engagement—and for the first time in my life I missed a connecting flight. I got the initial flight from London, no problem, but there was a long layover in Dubai. I was in the lounge, fell asleep, and on waking suddenly ran the entire length of the airport to the departure gate, only to find that they'd already closed the flight. What was frustrating was that the door to the air bridge was still open and I could see the plane, but they wouldn't let me board.

So then I had to look for the next available flight, which turned out to be twelve hours later, but on a different airline. No matter what happened, I had to be in Singapore by 7am on the Thursday to play golf with the organisers of an event. The original plan had been to arrive the night before. I called the organisers and told them what had happened. 'No problem— just get here whenever you can.' They were very reasonable and understanding. So I booked the flight and endured a fourteen-hour wait in Dubai before I flew to Singapore, arriving just in time to go directly to the golf course. I was already pretty exhausted and it wasn't going to get any easier.

After the golf, I finally made it to my hotel around 4pm, whereupon I met a business colleague for drinks prior to going on to a dinner with some friends. I got back to the hotel around midnight. I was up again the next morning to play more golf in the steamy Singapore heat, prior to yet another drinks function. You're probably thinking, 'What's he complaining about? Playing golf, going out for drinks—in Singapore', but I'm just trying to get across that there was a lot going on and I was short of sleep. Saturday was clear until the evening, when I was due to address five hundred or so people at a rugby club charity dinner.

The dinner over, I tried late on Saturday night to check in to my flight to Brisbane the next day, and to my horror discovered that my entire onward itinerary had been cancelled. Apparently, as soon as you don't show up for a specific flight— as I hadn't while snoring away in the Dubai executive lounge— all your ongoing legs are automatically cancelled. So I spent all night trying to organise a flight to Australia. Finally I contacted a friend who was high up in the airline and they agreed to get me on a flight and waive all extra costs.

I departed the next day and arrived very early in the morning in Brisbane. That afternoon I played golf with my father at Royal Queensland Golf Club—and for someone who'd been in three different countries and barely slept for four days, I played pretty well.

IAN LYNAGH: Michael arrived at around 6am in Brisbane and, as usual, Marie and I went to pick him up. Michael seems to enjoy coming home. We had some breakfast and went over to the golf course where I'd organised a game with a couple of friends of mine. Michael was quiet and he looked tired. He always pushes himself. He didn't want any dinner and then he insisted that he'd walk to the bar where he was due to meet his friends in the evening. We may have made the comment that he was having a pretty tiring day by doing everything he'd done then going out at night.

Prior to leaving for Australia, I had written to a couple of the guys I commonly kept in touch with, saying, 'Let's go out and have a beer.'

There were two groups that I met with in Brisbane from time to time. The first was mainly school friends and the second was university friends and guys I'd played rugby with over the years. Because of my TV commitments, I'd been in New Zealand for the 2011 World Cup, which meant I'd missed the previous year's informal gatherings, so I was extra keen to catch up with friends on this occasion. They were all busy guys doing different things and whenever I came over they would say, 'Mate, this is great. You give us a reason to get together.'

So I'd told the guys I was going to be in town and we'd arranged to assemble the two groups on successive nights. The first group agreed to meet on my first night at home, the Monday night, at 6.30pm at a place called Friday's, a club owned by a friend of mine, down by the river in the CBD area of Brisbane. It's a really nice spot. There's a beautiful deck and it was meant to be a relaxing evening with friends: steak, a couple of beers and some good-humoured chat. We certainly did not have plans for a big night.

We met as arranged, and started talking as a group of male friends usually does—telling a few old stories from the past. Well, just as I was taking a sip of my XXXX beer, a mate of mine, Peter Hancock, delivered the punchline of his story.

The joke went down well; my beer didn't.

Immediately I started coughing uncontrollably.

We've all done it when a drink goes down the wrong way, but this was more than normally forceful and violent. It took me a few seconds afterwards to catch my breath. I stopped coughing, gathered myself and then when I finally opened my eyes, I couldn't focus. I could see vague shapes and colour but nothing more detailed than that. I was also very dizzy.

PETER HANCOCK, SCHOOL FRIEND: The night started out as per usual: a group of mates sitting around having something to eat, a few beers and exchanging stories. Noddy was sitting at the head of the table and I was sitting to his immediate left. I recall telling a humorous story from our younger days. As I delivered the punchline I remember hearing Noddy start coughing as if his beer had gone down the wrong way. After a period of time (I don't know how long), Noddy said that he couldn't see to his left-hand side. He seemed fairly calm. At first I thought he was taking the piss.

I sat there shaking my head for a second to see if I could regain focus. I was even composed enough to quickly analyse the likely cause and to conclude that it was probably a combination of jetlag, general tiredness and a momentary lack of oxygen caused by the cough.

I thought, 'It'll come back.'

But it didn't come back.

At that moment I knew that there was something not right. Over forty-something years of relying on and listening to my body, I'd become pretty tuned in to when issues were serious—and this was something completely unlike anything I'd ever felt before. It was a really weird sensation and I could also feel a blinding headache starting to develop. It was an all-encompassing pain.

Having said all that, I could still feel and I could talk—I was still in the game, so to speak, but the lack of vision on my left side was really starting to scare me. Strangely, even then, the word 'stroke' never entered my mind, although I later heard that Peter Hancock had whispered, 'I think he might be having a stroke.'

Regardless, the details of the next few minutes are very hazy for me. Originally I thought that I was lying down for much of the time. To this day I have no idea why I thought that. But I was later told that I was sitting on my chair and able to talk quite lucidly.

PETER HANCOCK: I think because Noddy wanted us to call an ambulance, we all thought it was serious. I can't speak for the others, but I was very concerned, having been through a similar ordeal with my wife, Angie.

Ironically, an old school friend of mine, John Matson, who had travelled down from the north coast for the get-together, had literally just left. John is a GP. That left Tony McNamee—a physiotherapist and the only one of the remaining group with any kind of medical qualification—to ask, 'Are you okay, mate?'

'Give me a moment,' I said.

I shook my head again to try and shift the fog. Nothing changed.

Then Tony said, 'Shall we call an ambulance?'

I said yes immediately.

Sometimes you just know what's needed. This was one of those times. You don't second-guess that kind of instinct. I suppose I was hoping that they'd put me in an ambulance, take me to the hospital and fix it all there and then. Tony also asked me if I wanted him to call my parents and again I said yes. I had my phone in my pocket and I was able to get it out, remember the four-digit security code and tell Tony how to scroll through the menus to access my parents' phone number—he had to because I don't know my parents' number by heart. I don't even know my own number by heart.

When the paramedics arrived—and they did so pretty rapidly—I was able to walk, with some assistance, down the steps of the club to the ambulance, but I have no recollection of the journey to hospital, probably because—I'm told—they immediately started to administer oxygen and possibly some painkillers to keep me comfortable.

IAN LYNAGH: We got a call from Tony McNamee around 9.45pm saying that Michael had had a bad headache and couldn't see … and that they'd called an ambulance as a precaution. My immediate thought was that maybe he'd had a bad migraine. A headache and vision issues? Migraine seemed the most likely explanation. Where we live is between the restaurant and the hospital and as we got ready and jumped in the car, we actually heard the ambulance going past at the end of the road. When we arrived at the hospital, Tony McNamee and another member of the group, Steven Grant, were sitting in the waiting room. At that point the ambulance had not arrived and then, shortly afterwards, we saw the ambulance pull in. We had no idea of the seriousness at this point. We still thought that he was tired, had overdone it a little maybe, which was a stupid diagnosis when you look back on it, but at that early stage nobody really knew what was wrong.

Whatever happened after my arrival at the Royal Brisbane Hospital is mostly unclear to me. I have only fuzzy, sketchy recollections of who was there, what was said and when. Despite being given some kind of pain-relieving medication, I do remember registering that the headache was still very much there. The pain was totally debilitating.

I also remember vaguely noting that the situation was being taken very seriously. It was a feeling in the air. Even in my dazed state I could feel the urgency and energy in the acute care unit, and the fact that Rob Henderson—head of the neurology department—was called at home also seemed indicative of the seriousness.

I should say that I knew very little about stroke. It wasn't something I'd ever thought about and it had certainly never crossed my mind that I could have one. As far as I was concerned, stroke was something that affected older people or those with very unhealthy lifestyles. I fell into neither of those categories. I was fit for my age, still went to the gym regularly and ate reasonably healthily. I liked a glass of wine once in a while, but who doesn't? It was going to take a while to come to terms with the fact that I'd just had a major stroke at the age of forty-eight.

DR ROBERT HENDERSON, CONSULTANT NEUROLOGIST: I was at home when I received a phone call late at night from my on-duty staff saying simply that they had a 48-year-old ex-footie player admitted with symptoms that might suggest an acute stroke. They wanted me to have a look at the scans. No mention of a name. Now, at that time of an evening, there's every chance that the staff who were working were probably (a) fairly young and (b) predominantly from overseas, so only when I arrived at the hospital did I realise that this wasn't just any ex-footie player. Of course, being from Brisbane and also being in my forties, I knew exactly who Michael Lynagh was.

The priority for the acute medical staff when someone is admitted with symptoms like mine is to establish the cause as quickly as possible—ideally within the first hour of admission. It's a very critical stage in the treatment of stroke because, with the blood vessels still potentially unstable, the risk of another stroke is still very high. A second stroke could have meant devastating damage.

With that in mind, the first step is usually to take a CT perfusion scan to establish what's causing the symptoms, as well as to highlight what damage has already been done. I don't recall the scan itself but I do remember the confirmation I received from the head neurologist, Rob Henderson, that the right (the human body has two) vertebral artery at the back of my head had dissected, causing a blood clot which in turn led to a large stroke in what was initially thought to be two areas of my brain.

DR HENDERSON: There is a system in place whereby anyone admitted to the emergency area with symptoms suggestive of acute stroke could be given a procedure called thrombolysis within an hour of arrival. Thrombolysis is designed to dissolve blood clots in cases of acute stroke and it involves the introduction of thrombolytic drugs. When I arrived at the hospital, Michael had already had a CT perfusion scan. That scan is designed to distinguish areas of brain tissue that can be salvaged by thrombolysis from those areas that will go into infarct, or, in everyday terms, a state of tissue death. What was extremely positive was that Michael was outwardly quite healthy: his scan pictures looked much worse than he did. He was very with it and able to talk so we were able to get a clear history from him. The results of the CT perfusion scan, however, ruled thrombolysis out because it was clear to me from the images I was seeing that the stroke was not, in this case, reversible.

The major problem for Michael was actually in a different part of his brain from where it first appeared. It first appeared that the part of the brain that controls vision—the occipital lobe—was the major problem. Although it did, in the long run, turn out to be the major issue, the bigger problem at this early stage was damage to his cerebellum—the area of the brain that controls coordination. That damage had not been too obvious initially, but for the first three days after a stroke there's a major risk of swelling [to the cerebellum].

Rob Henderson explained to my parents and me that the artery that had dissected was at that moment largely stable and, in fact, had blocked itself off with a clot at the initial stage, and then that block would hopefully later be reinforced by scar tissue. It scared me to think that this was actually going on in my head. But the fact that the artery was blocked was good news. If it doesn't block off, there's the risk of more blood leaking through to push upwards and dislodge another clot that could lead to further strokes. In some cases, if the artery doesn't block off, surgeons can go in and surgically seal it off, but in my case that wasn't necessary.

IAN LYNAGH: We were outside in the hallway talking to a couple of the specialists and at that point things seemed a little more serious. Across the hallway was a glass office where all the doctors and emergency crew were. Coincidentally, from where I was sitting, I could see an x-ray they'd put up on the screen. I said to Marie: 'Jeez, that poor guy's in a bit of trouble.' I could see a big blob at the base of the occipital area—it was the size of a fist, maybe even bigger. 'I hope to God that's not Michael's brain,' I went on to add. Not for a single second did I think it was, but, as it turned out, that's exactly what I was looking at. We waited for another fifteen minutes and then a group—including Rob Henderson—came to talk to us. I don't recall a lot of the information he gave us at the time. I was still in shock.

MARIE LYNAGH: By this time Michael had given me all his personal possessions—his wallet, keys and phone—but before we left for the night, he insisted that I give him his phone so he could call Isabella. I told him that he wasn't allowed to call from the emergency area. 'I don't care. I have to call Isabella,' he said. And he did. The other thing he was very concerned about was his commitments to Sky Sports that weekend, so we agreed that we'd call them first thing the following morning to explain what had happened.

After I spoke to Isabella that night, I felt a little more relaxed. The call was definitely emotional—it's a phone call that nobody ever wants to have to make. Despite the dire situation I was in, my aim was to assure her that I was in the best possible place. 'I'll be fine. The doctors know what they're doing—just focus on the boys,' I said.

I was already pretty certain that I didn't want her to drop everything and fly to Australia. I actually felt it might hinder my recovery, as I'd be worrying about where the family would stay and the fact that the boys were missing school. Also, there really wasn't much they could do. I thought that it was more important for Isabella and the boys to maintain their routine. I also didn't want to send a negative message to the boys. It was hard to do, but I wanted to make a mature decision for everyone's sake. I thought that to panic and fly Isabella and the kids out would have made it seem as if I was preparing to see them for the last time. I thought that would be a knee-jerk reaction. Weak. I was more interested in maintaining, as far as possible, a degree of normality in a 'Dad's going to be fine' kind of way.

ISABELLA LYNAGH: I was actually under a bit of pressure from some friends that were saying: 'What are you doing? Your husband is in hospital. You go, we'll look after the kids.' It started to get to me after a while. I was talking to Michael and we had discussed what the best thing to do was. I was acting on his wishes—what we both thought was best for all of us. It proved to be the right decision.

I wanted to transmit to Isabella and the boys a sense that the situation was under control, even if it wasn't. I always think that there are certain things children need to be shielded from, to some degree, and me being in hospital in a critical condition, thousands of miles away, was definitely one of them. Their feelings were much more important than mine at that moment.

ISABELLA LYNAGH: Michael was obviously heavily sedated, but he was still very lucid. He told me what happened, about choking on the beer and that he had this big headache. He also told me that he couldn't see very well. He was very reassuring and I think that's one of the reasons I kept my sanity. It's in Michael's nature to play things down sometimes and he does that so that I don't worry too much. He just wanted everything at home to be calm and for us to carry on as normal. Michael actually spoke to me every day while he was in hospital. He doesn't remember that, but he did.

The following morning was when the full enormity of what had happened dawned on me. My parents and I met with Rob Henderson and Craig Winter, another of the senior neurologists. They showed us the scan images and explained exactly what they meant. Rob pointed to a large area of swelling at the base of my skull, very close to my brain stem. It wasn't good news.

In addition to the small area of stroke around my right vertebral artery that was causing the loss of vision on my left side (the medical term is hemiopia), there was another area of even greater concern. A separate part of my brain—the cerebellum—was also showing significant stroke damage. It's the part of the brain that controls coordination and it was this section that had swollen and was at risk from further swelling.

It was a major worry. The already swollen cerebellum was fractions of millimetres away from pressing down on my brain stem, and if that happened the results would be catastrophic. I was likely to die, the surgeons said.

Die?

That word really hit me hard.

I guess I just wasn't ready to confront my mortality so suddenly. Are you ever ready? The severity of my situation didn't seem real, because of how able I was and felt. There I was, I'd survived a massive stroke when others often don't, but there was still a possibility that I might not survive. That possibility was hard to fathom.

ISABELLA LYNAGH: Michael's mum rang me and said, 'Isabella, this could all go very badly, very shortly.' She explained to me about the swelling and that really freaked me out. I couldn't comprehend how serious it was because I'd been talking to him and he seemed fine. My best friend told me later that she saw me crying outside school the day Marie called. I tried to stay strong. Completely losing it, with my husband in a critical condition in Australia and me stuck in England with the kids, wouldn't have helped anybody. So I tried to stay strong for everyone. I knew it was the right thing for me not to fly to Brisbane. Part of me knew he'd make it.

In 1993, when he was sick with peritonitis, I remember his dad ringing me and saying he was in a really bad way. My feeling was, again, 'It just can't end this way.' Our relationship had started so magically and I had a really strong belief that this was not the way the story was going to end. I kept telling him to stay strong.

I even lay in bed at night, consciously sending all my positive energy his way.

So what were the available options?

Well, brain surgery was one that was discussed as a possible means of easing the dangerous swelling. Apparently the surgery is reasonably standard; Rob Henderson said that in a normal week he might conduct that kind of operation three or four times. But invasive surgery of any kind always carries with it a certain degree of risk. The fact that the organ involved was the brain merely added to that risk. It was the specialist's job to weigh up the pros and cons.

'Oh my God,' I remember thinking when brain surgery was mentioned. 'This really is a pretty serious thing.'

A section of skull at the back of my head would have to be removed (and not replaced)—hardly a pleasant procedure—but the alternative outcome of the swelling continuing just didn't bear consideration. What was in my favour was that—despite the size and severity of the stroke—I was still functioning very well. Rob Henderson was very surprised by that. I was alert; I could talk. So the discussion was based around the fact that I was arguably functioning too well to risk surgical intervention to reduce the swelling. But one way or another, that swelling had to be addressed quickly.

It was a surreal feeling, sitting there, thinking about what was going on. I remember suddenly feeling the urge to ask my mother: 'Is the corner of my mouth drooping?' I'd once read that that was one of the first outwardly obvious symptoms stroke victims experience. I was relieved to be told that it wasn't, but to ask that question at such a stressful moment was indicative of my determination, which would develop throughout the recovery process: a need to confirm and check off, as if from a list, abilities that I had before the stroke, to confirm that I still had them. Yes, my vision was affected, but everything else, miraculously, seemed to be untouched.

IAN LYNAGH: In that first conversation with Rob Henderson, I asked him, 'If we're not doing brain surgery, what's the other alternative?' 'Wait,' he said. 'Dehydrate him, pump him with medication and just wait.' I asked him what the prognosis of this treatment was and his answer still gives me chills today when I think about it. 'We don't know because they don't usually survive.'

When the doctors were sitting at the foot of my bed that morning, discussing all the options, I also felt a sense of resignation. I was absolutely terrified of brain surgery. What would I have left when I came out of it? Would I come out of it at all? But I was also conceding that it might be necessary. My thinking was, 'If this is what needs to be done to fix me, then this is what must be done. I'm ready to go.'

Bizarrely, when the invasive surgery option was ruled out, I didn't think, 'Thank goodness.' I actually thought, 'Why? If this is what's needed, why don't you just do it?'

Maybe I just wanted a quick fix. It was only when Rob Henderson explained the reasons again that I accepted that there was another option.

Based on what must have been a lot of consultation among themselves, the neurologists decided that the best course of action was to dehydrate me in an attempt to ease the swelling of the cerebellum. While the dehydration process was taking place—and it would take a few days—they'd monitor and wake me every thirty minutes to ensure that the swelling was indeed going in the right direction.

At each waking they would assess my ability to do various things—all of which would confirm to them that the process was effective. I was told that the next three days were absolutely critical for my recovery. It was explained to me as being similar to what happens with a very bad ankle sprain. It's initially painful, but then the worst swelling comes in days two to five. Then the swelling eases. That's what would happen to my brain, but the consequences of that swelling not going down would be far more serious.

As strange and utterly irrelevant as it might sound, one of the issues that was bugging me was my commitment to Sky that weekend. I was due back in the studio on Saturday morning to cover the Heineken Cup. I also had a meeting with a bank on the following Monday. I desperately didn't want to let anybody down and it was pretty obvious to me that I wasn't going to be there. So I asked Mum and Dad to call Fitzy at Sky and the bank representative as soon as possible to let them know what was happening. It was vitally important to me.

SEAN 'FITZY' FITZPATRICK, MICHAEL'S CO-COMMENTATOR AT SKY: I was in Marrakech, Morocco, when I got a phone call from Michael's father. It was early in the morning. He told me what had happened—I hadn't heard from anyone else. I was shocked like everyone was. Ian told me that Michael was worried about not being back in the studio that Saturday. I wasn't really surprised by that. That's how Michael is. I just said, 'Tell him not to even give it a thought.' In the grand scheme of things it just wasn't important.

FOURTEEN

THE LOWEST EBB

DR HENDERSON: The first three days after stroke are critical for two reasons. Firstly, the artery in question is still considered unstable and further stroke can occur—leading to a devastating outcome. Secondly, the stroke that had already occurred in the cerebellum (the less obviously affected area, initially) was at major risk of swelling. Michael was within a whisker of having that part of his brain removed surgically—which isn't an unusual procedure—but he needed to get through this initial risk period. What we'd be looking at over these few days would be for the artery to not change when we examined with follow-up imaging. In Michael's case, we were more hopeful of stabilisation because it was blocked off. Once it's blocked off, it doesn't have that pressure pushing upwards with the potential to dislodge a piece of blood clot. And once a clot dislodges there's nowhere for it to go other than to kill brain tissue.

IN MY ALREADY SLEEP-DEPRIVED state, being woken every half-hour for routine observations wasn't pleasant. The nurses would ask me a series of questions designed to test my faculties.

They wanted to see if I could come up with the right answers every time. Changes in my responses, or my ability to think logically, could give clues to life-threatening issues going on inside my brain. I was on a strict thirty-minute schedule, like a prisoner on suicide watch.

'Who's the prime minister of Australia?'

'What's the date?'

'What's your sister's name?'

'What's *your* name?'

I knew what date it was because it was around the time of my son Thomas's birthday, so I could add a day or two to figure that out. I knew who the prime minister was but then they'd ask me who the *previous* prime minister was ...

The question I could never get my head around was when they asked what ward of the hospital I was in. I never seemed to be able to get the words 'intensive care' out. I used to say, 'Oh, I know it's three letters', or 'It's somewhere you go when you're really sick', or maybe I'd say 'Emergency.'

'You mean the ICU?'

'Yeah, that's it!'

For some reason I just couldn't remember it.

Then they'd ask me to grab their hands with both hands to assess whether I still had strength. Or to lift my legs and push down to show that I could still do that. This process went on every half-hour for two days solid. It was absolutely exhausting, and a lot of the time I did it almost automatically, with my eyes closed. I knew what was coming and that in itself must have been a good sign for the medical staff.

With the continual comings and goings, all day every day, the ICU area of a major hospital isn't the easiest place to sleep at the best of times. I remember a woman came in at one point, screaming and yelling at the top of her voice. I don't know what was wrong with her but she definitely wasn't in a good way. Then a guy came in who'd been in a serious car accident. That wasn't pretty either.

There was a constant cacophony of noise and almost all of it was indicative of pain and upset. After all, by definition, the intensive care unit exists to deal with the worst cases—those that need urgent medical attention—and some of what I saw and heard in there has been hard to forget. I still don't understand how the hospital staff do what they do. They are heroes. They see horrific things every single day and they just have to deal with it. Maybe they detach themselves somehow from the fact that it's real human beings they're seeing in awful situations.

Consequently, those two or three days and nights post-stroke included some of the toughest moments I've ever experienced. I say 'days and nights', but in reality there was no obvious difference between night and day for me at that time. It was all just *time*—hour upon indistinguishable hour of freezing cold, headaches and exhaustion on a level I'd never felt before. In addition, the process of dehydration was pretty mind-boggling. The volume of fluid that left my body was staggering—there were literally buckets of it. It was pouring out of me, taking any strength I had left with it. There was also a balance to be struck between dehydrating me sufficiently to reduce the swelling in my brain, and leaving me with enough fluid to stay alive. That's one of the main reasons why I was in the intensive care unit: so my levels of hydration could be carefully observed.

There was a lot of medical activity going on during these initial few days and much of it involved needles. I don't like needles—never have done. And I was getting a lot of them poked into me as part of the administering of medication and blood tests. Eventually I said, 'I hate this. There's got to be another way.' My arms were starting to look like a drug addict's.

Thankfully, there was a viable alternative. Instead of having to inject me all the time, the doctors wanted to insert a cannula into my arm so that they could administer drugs that way. The thought of that didn't thrill me, though, and because I was already nervous my veins collapsed as soon as the staff tried to put anything in. They tried at least three times to get the cannula into my left arm—they just couldn't do it. At the moment the staff switched over to my right arm to try a vein there, my father walked in. There was a doctor hunched over me, and blood everywhere. I think Dad must have thought, 'Oh jeez, he's gone and slashed his wrists.' It was a bloody mess. Eventually they managed to get the cannula situated, but it was a struggle.

LOUIS LYNAGH, MICHAEL'S ELDEST SON: When my mum first told us, I was just about to go to school. Mum told us what had happened to Dad and we were all frightened. I remember thinking about what we'd all do if he didn't make it. Some of the teachers at school had heard about it and they asked, 'Are you all right?' They were all very nice to me. All I could do was keep hoping that he'd get better quickly and come home again.

WEDNESDAY WAS THE DAY when things got really difficult. I was just too tired; I hadn't eaten or slept properly for three days and the pain in my head was unbearable. Additionally, the process of dehydration was exacerbating my gout, from which

I'd suffered for some time. I guess the uric acid had nothing to dilute it. The pain was excruciating—in my feet and my knee. I wasn't allowed to take my normal medication. It was absolute agony.

It was at this time that a good friend of mine—an architect, Mick Hellen—came in to visit me with my parents. I was in no state whatsoever to have visitors. I seem to remember being told that Mick had brought me chewing gum. Mick's a top bloke but I realised as he was chatting away that he had no concept of how serious this was. Somehow that made everything seem even more serious to me.

IAN LYNAGH: Mick wanted to come and visit Michael and he brought a pile of surfing magazines for him to read. I remember thinking that there was just no way that Michael was ready for that. He [Mick] had no idea how serious it was. Mick's a lovely, easygoing guy and, after he'd been there for a while, Michael said: 'Dad, I'm sorry, but do you mind asking him to leave? I need to talk to you.' Of course, Mick understood.

When Mick left, I asked Mum to leave the room too and beckoned Dad to come closer to me. My mood had darkened. Like clouds, negative thoughts had rolled in and wouldn't stop coming. My resolve was weakening. I was starting to doubt whether I was going to make it. I was too tired, too sore, too cold. They tried everything to warm me up, even putting space-blankets on me at one point, but I felt like I was freezing to death.

I thought about some of the toughest moments I'd spent on a rugby field—pulling victory from defeat in the last few minutes in Dublin, winning at Eden Park in '86, overcoming other people's injuries to defeat Natal in Durban to win the 1994 Super 10 for Queensland. All these moments flashed through my head in agonising slow motion, like that heart-wrenching highlight reel at the end of the Italian movie *Cinema Paradiso*. Only now it was me watching my own life, with just the sound of an imaginary projector breaking the silence. I saw all the faces of everyone dear to me: Isabella; the boys; my parents; my sister, Jane—where were they now? I *needed* them now ...

I wasn't sure how much more I could take. It seemed too hard to fight. I was ready to not see my wife again, not see the boys grow up. I actually thought about it practically—what it would really mean. Weighed it all up. And I still came to the conclusion that it was just too hard a battle. It sounds weak now, but I'm being completely honest about how I felt. I can't deny it.

It was my lowest moment ever. And I just couldn't seem to turn it around. I'd often read about people in dire situations who are faced with the 'Do I have the strength to keep going?' question. As an observer I used to think, 'Oh, come on, surely nothing is so bad that you can't get through it?'

But I can assure you, as strong as your mind is (and I'd always thought mine was), if you're worn down physically to absolute breaking point, you just can't predict what kind of decisions you'll find yourself making. Not in a million years did I ever think I'd say, 'It's easier to give up', but here I was, about to do it. I was succumbing.

I remember that I asked Dad to get a paper towel from beside the sink and said, 'Look Dad, in case I don't survive, I want you to write these details down.' Mentally, I'd just crossed another line. It's one thing thinking certain thoughts, but it's another thing entirely when you take practical steps based on what you're thinking.

I had bank accounts that only I knew the passwords to. And my worry was that they might never be found once I was gone. Isabella didn't know about these accounts; I'd never told her. It wasn't that I'd been secretive or had ever thought of hiding anything from her. It was just that I'd lived in three countries over the years and had a number of accounts and policies that she'd always been happy for me to manage for the benefit of all the family. But she would *need* to know, if I didn't survive. So I wanted Dad to jot down the information. 'Promise you'll make sure the boys are okay,' I asked him next. I was thinking about the future. Their future. The boys were young. They had school fees due, university to pay for after that, holidays to go on, first cars to buy, weddings—all the things I'd never see them do. All these things I'd never be a part of.

I felt no self-pity, only exhaustion. And pain. At that moment I fully accepted that I was going to die in a hospital bed in Brisbane with my wife and kids in another country. No goodbyes, no hugs, no final 'We love you, Dad'.

I'd just be gone.

IAN LYNAGH: He wanted to give me these details. Nobody else knew them—that's typical of Michael. 'It's complex,' he said. So I wrote the information down. Then he said, 'Dad, I want you to promise me that you'll look after the boys.' I swallowed hard. Choked back tears. He was preparing to die—there's no other way of saying it. We both kept our composure there, but not so much at home.

When Dad left, I really didn't know if I'd see him again. I remember looking at the clock in the room: it was 7pm. I closed my eyes to relieve the pain, not knowing when or if I'd open them.

MARIE LYNAGH: When we got home that evening, Michael's story had obviously hit the press during that day. When I opened the door of the house, the phone was making this terrible noise. I called Telstra in the morning and they sent an engineer round. As I said my name he said, 'Oh, Michael Lynagh! Let me fix this straightaway.' It turned out that the phone had completely melted down from all the calls and messages that had been coming in during the day. The Telstra engineer just couldn't do enough for us.

FIFTEEN

THE TURNING POINT

I MUST HAVE FALLEN asleep …

I was in a place I'd been many times before, on the coast north of Brisbane. Buddina Beach, it's called, and it's a long way from being the best surf-break on the coast. But it's a beautiful place and there is the occasional wave. It was ten-thirty in the morning—a scorching-hot summer day. I was about to have my second surf of the day. My parents were on the beach relaxing, reading the paper.

It wasn't what you'd call 'big' that day, but there was a sandbank with a gutter behind it that was creating some nice, shoulder-high lefts. This other guy and I were sitting out there, a hundred and fifty metres from the beach. To this day I have no idea who he was. Blazing sunshine, boardshorts and a few easy waves to catch. 'You take that one, mate—that wave is yours.' It was that kind of day.

About five metres in front of us, this big fish came up and went down again. I noted its position and said, 'Jeez, I hope that was a dolphin.' This guy goes, 'Me too.' It was pretty normal to see dolphins out there. They'd swim around and then come up out of nowhere and give you a huge fright—they'd be literally two metres away from you. But this was a little further away and it swam with a smooth glide rather than a dolphin's head and tail breach. It looked a bit different from a dolphin too, but we thought nothing more of it.

There weren't that many people in the area—certainly no warning flags or lifeguards. They were a kilometre or so further down the beach. But the twenty or so people who were on the beach were now waving at us—'Hey, hey!'

We turned around and saw, in the gutter between the beach and us, a shark slicing up and down, obviously looking for food. It was big and was probably looking at us, thinking, 'Your move, guys.'

So we're stuck on a sandbank that's two metres deep and between us and the beach is a gutter that's also quite deep. And in that gutter is a hungry shark.

I thought, 'What the hell do we do?' In all my years of surfing, I'd never been in this situation. I'd never even seen a shark. We could see the lifeguards starting to run along the beach and just then it seemed as if the shark had disappeared. We thought it might have gone back out to the deeper water.

I had a decision to make. Do I sit it out? Or do I make a paddle for it through the gutter? It was a twenty- or thirty-metre stretch of deep water. Close enough that we could almost touch the other side. Far enough that we'd be in a bit of trouble if a large predator wanted a chunk out of us. It was possible that the shark had gone. There was also a decent chance that it was still in there.

It was one of those situations in life when you weigh up your options given the information at your disposal—'What do I *want* the outcome to be?' Then you just do it. So I jumped into the gutter on my board with my feet raised out of the water and paddled as smoothly and quietly across it as hard as I could, towards the lifeguards who, by that time, were speeding out to meet me in an inflatable dinghy. The other guy did the same. Of course I thought about getting chewed and of course I looked down for any sign of a dark shadow flitting below me. But all the time I thought, 'I'm getting to that beach.'

As I was walking up the beach towards my parents, the noise of the sea disappeared and the vivid colours of that summer day faded.

I WOKE UP WITH a jolt—'This *is* real, after all.'

I wasn't on Buddina Beach anymore. I knew that because I was freezing cold. Every one of the four blankets I had wrapped tightly around me was in place, but I couldn't seem to retain any heat. The bed was wet. Soaking wet. I thought, 'I *can't* have peed the bed, can I?' That would have been embarrassing. That still mattered. Then I sensed that the bedclothes were soaked through with my sweat.

I lay there, unable to move. It must have been late at night because I sensed, through my tightly closed eyelids, that it was pitch black. I'd discovered that if I kept my eyes shut, some parts of me hurt less. Whenever I opened them, it seemed that my body was pained by the fact that the left side of my vision was missing. It was like emerging from total darkness into bright sunlight: there's a period of adjustment. It hurts. But there seemed to be no way of easing the pain in the back of my head. It was always there. Relentless.

As I lay still, trying to fall asleep again, I started to notice the noises of the machines around me in ICU. I hadn't really registered them before; during the day they were probably drowned out by all the other noise. One would bleep; then, a few seconds later, another would chime. Then another. They weren't the same tone or the same pitch; they came from completely different sources. But gradually, it seemed to me that they were connected. I almost smiled—'Surely, this can't be right?'

In my strange, semi-dazed state, I came to the conclusion that I was hearing the flute intro to the Canned Heat song 'Going up the Country'. I quite like that song. And it's pretty distinctive; most people know it. At no point did I ask myself what might seem to you to be the obvious question: 'How could a few pieces of medical equipment possibly combine to play a tune?' I just accepted it for what it was. It seemed perfectly plausible at that moment. So I leaned over and wrote two words on a piece of paper on my nightstand: 'Canned Heat'. I still have that piece of paper.

I fell asleep again, but this time I didn't dream. There was nothing but deep impenetrable black. The sleep the dead might sleep. But I wasn't dead. And then, however much later, when I woke up, it was almost as if a switch had been flipped down there in the blackness. I still felt exhausted, cold and in unbearable pain. That hadn't changed. The physical aspect was the same, and would continue to be for some days yet. But mentally—having been reminded of something from my real life, of something that existed outside the walls of the intensive care unit, of something from the days when I was healthy and happy—I felt a huge rush of positivity. It wasn't 'I'll hang on for a bit longer', or 'Maybe I can beat this.' It was far more emphatic than that.

'I'm *going* to see my kids again.'

It was a moment of monumental clarity.

IAN LYNAGH: When we came in on the Thursday morning, Michael seemed like a totally different person. His attitude had changed, seemingly overnight. We'd told our daughter, Jane, whose birthday it had recently been, how bad Michael was the night before and she'd come up from Sydney to see him. Michael was brighter and seemed ready to get on with his life. Almost as if he'd decided, 'This is a new day; I'm going to fight this.' Medically he wasn't out of the woods, but mentally he seemed to be.

As soon as my mental state turned around, my physical condition responded in kind. It was a slow process, obviously, but it was one that I knew was in motion. I had a scan on the Friday morning and the doctors told me that the swelling on my brain was gradually receding. I could almost feel it contracting, finally relieving the pressure.

My sister, Jane, came to visit me later that morning. Despite the fact that we had never been particularly close, she was incredibly emotional when she saw me—she seemed genuinely pleased that I was alive! As she was leaving, she started crying again. I'm not entirely sure why. In hindsight, I think it was just her way of showing her relief and happiness, but at the time it seemed as if she might be wondering if she'd ever see me again. I comforted her and told her, 'Don't worry,

Jane, I'm not going anywhere.' I knew I wasn't going anywhere but home.

AS A RESULT OF my improvement, Rob Henderson and the team decided to move me from ICU to the general ward on Sunday, where the Acute Rehab team would monitor my eyesight and my coordination. It was a significant step towards recovery. The hospital gave me a room on my own in the ward because they figured I'd have a lot of visitors. It was quite comfortable, with a bathroom adjoining. It felt like I'd been upgraded to first class. There was also a small television set. It got me thinking.

My biggest worry was my eyesight. Rob Henderson had explained that the damaged artery had caused irreparable damage to areas of my brain called the occipital lobe and the lateral medulla. The occipital lobe is the part that affects eyesight and the damage to its right side was causing what's called contralateral issues with my vision on the left side. As far as I could understand, that damage was permanent. But the stroke that affected part of my lateral medulla had caused no noticeable issues.

I kept saying to myself, 'What am I going to be able to see?' I was worried about things like reading and watching TV—all the things that I had taken for granted before I lost a significant part of my field of vision on the left side. Those had always seemed such simple things. Now I was forced to re-evaluate my capabilities. I needed to know particularly if I'd be able to continue my work with Sky, which involved watching a screen for long periods.

First I picked up a magazine and thought, 'I can read!' There were some issues in that I couldn't see the entire page, but I could read. Then I turned on the little portable hospital TV—'I can watch it!' I quickly realised that small TVs were going to be easier than wide ones, though. My reduced field of vision meant that I could see all of a small screen, but only part of a large one. The left side would be missing if I was looking directly at the middle of a large screen. Regardless, it was a big thrill that I could see at all.

ALAN JONES: I was keeping in contact with Michael's parents on a daily basis throughout. I wanted to mention him on my radio show that goes out across Australia. But I was wary of saying anything publicly on the radio that would compromise his privacy. But at an appropriate time, he told me that it was appropriate for me to say the things that I said, and to outline what happened. Lo and behold, Ross Reynolds—a member of that same Grand Slam team—had been listening to my broadcast. Not long after that, in the presence of his wife, he faced similar circumstances, and it was because she recognised the circumstances I'd described about Michael's situation that she raced her husband to the doctor. He, too, had had a stroke and he, too, was saved.

That night, lying in my bed, I began to think about going to the toilet. I hadn't been eating (I'd immediately thrown up the first bit of food I'd tried) but I had been taking in a little fluid as the swelling on my brain slowly decreased. Technically, I was meant to call a nurse for assistance, but I started wondering if I could do it myself.

I was testing myself. Finding my measure. I've always needed a measure.

'Okay, I've established that I can see. But can I walk?' I had to know. But I didn't want to fall and set my recovery back. Or get in trouble with the nurses.

I lay there, surveying the room in detail. I made mental notes of potential supports and handholds: a corner of a nightstand, the edge of a wardrobe. I also identified a few obvious risks: a curtain or a lamp cable to trip on. Finally, I looked for escape routes: 'If I fall there, I can grab onto this …' It felt like an assault course. 'Can I get there?' I wondered. It would be a matter of sheer will.

DR HENDERSON: Michael was a great case of when you should treat the patient, not the scan. The whole way through, Michael's coordination had been pretty much intact. I've told him that his cerebellum must be a bit different from the average person's. Even though he lost a fair bit of it, he was born with a better cerebellum than most people. Your coordination for walking, in particular, is affected in that area, but in his case he was untouched. Michael didn't know this at the time, but there was also a tiny area of stroke—a third area—close to his brain stem. It barely showed up in the initial scans. At one stage we sent him down again and asked them to do some particularly fine cuts on the scanner, right through a particular area on his brain stem, and we were fairly satisfied that there had been some stroke damage, but it wasn't a big deal.

I swung my legs over the side of the bed and stood unassisted for the first time in over a week. I wasn't totally stable, but at no point did I feel that I'd fall, either. Gradually, I picked my way across the room, using the previously noted aids on the way and avoiding the hazards. I felt like I was in a video game. I made it, and the return journey was successful too. Back in bed I thought to myself, 'I can do this. I'm on the way back.'

MARIE LYNAGH: When we came in on the Saturday morning, Michael was elated. He told us that he had managed to get to the bathroom unaided and it really seemed like he saw that as a huge obstacle that he'd overcome. It was monumental. Now he wanted to walk. So he got out of bed and walked, slowly at first, in a straight line to the end of the ward and back.

Having managed to get to the bathroom, I felt that I was ready to try to walk properly. Nobody else thought that, but Rob and the specialists couldn't really argue with my progress. It seemed I was completely defying the odds. Rob said, 'You shouldn't really be able to do any of this. This is very unusual.'

The next morning, just after Mum had arrived to visit, I decided that I was going to walk to the end of the ward and back in a perfectly straight line. Mum was reluctant to let me try, but I was determined, as painful as my feet still were from gout, to prove to myself that I could.

I stood up and was instantly reminded that I had absolutely no strength. It was hardly a surprise, given how the last week had played out: a stroke, very little sleep and almost no food. But I did have coordination. I was almost conscious of trying to send the signal from my brain to my limbs, and my nervous system worked as it always had; the signals were getting through. I was elated. I thought to myself, 'I've had a stroke but I can read, watch TV, walk ...'

IAN LYNAGH: One of the signs that I got that the real Michael was back was when I arrived one day as he was being taken downstairs for physiotherapy. There was a wheelchair sitting there for him and I said, 'Come on, Mike, I'll push you down.' Well he turned to me and said, 'I'm not getting in that.' He was actually irritated. He insisted on walking on his own to the elevator. He wouldn't let me help him at all. I thought to myself, 'He's getting normal.'

AS PART OF MY rehabilitation process, they started taking me downstairs to the physiotherapy department every morning. I looked forward to it. It was a chance to measure my progress. I was enjoying getting stronger and being able to do some of the exercises the physio showed me.

But, more significantly, I was realising that the physical side of my recovery was very important, just as important as my mental breakthrough. I wondered if it was because I was an ex-athlete and had been in good condition for my age before the stroke. Maybe knowing what it was to be very fit and healthy made me want to do everything I could to get back? That was certainly how it seemed and my actions seemed to confirm it.

The physios put me through a series of balance tests: walking upstairs, balancing on one leg and then balancing on the other leg. Some of the tests had a visual element built in. They asked me to step off a low platform to establish how well I could see the differential between the platform and the floor. I suppose it simulated stepping off a footpath—the kind of challenge I'd soon be facing in the outside world. Then the physios would ask me to walk through sand to test my balance. I could do everything at the level of a normally functioning person. Nobody could understand why. But to me it was the least I expected of myself. I thought, 'Why shouldn't I be able to do this?'

IAN LYNAGH: Michael got through the tests pretty much like a 'normal' person. [His actions were] far less [like those of] a person who'd just had a major stroke, some of it affecting the part of his brain that controlled limb coordination. There was no actual strength there, but he was able to move exactly as they wanted him to.

As the next few days passed, my mood improved consistently. I started to get regular visits from friends who wanted to see me: Slacky, Helmet, Alan Jones—all kinds of people I realised I hadn't seen in person for many years. But nothing had changed. Five minutes of talking and we were right back as if we were on tour, in the dressing room or on the golf course together.

PETER HANCOCK: Tony McNamee and I visited him on the following Sunday. We were expecting him to be laid up in bed in his hospital gown. We walked into his room and there he was in his jeans, button-up shirt and deck shoes, looking like a million bucks! Andrew Slack came in about five minutes later and the four of us sat around shooting the breeze. Noddy was sitting there chatting away as if nothing had happened – unbelievable.

It was extremely moving to see my old friends, and I registered how lucky I was to have so many good ones. Rugby is like that. When someone needs help, people come out of the woodwork to give their support.

TIM HORAN: I went in to see Noddy and by that time you wouldn't have known he'd had a stroke. He had ice on his feet and I said, 'If you had a stroke, why have you got ice on your feet, mate?' We had a laugh about that. The consultant came in while I was there and I remember him saying to Michael, 'You've not dodged a bullet here; you've dodged a cannonball.' At that moment, from joking about his feet, I realised how lucky we were to still have Noddy with us.

THE DAY BEFORE I left hospital, one of the nurses came over to Mum, who was with me at the time, and said, 'What do we do with all the cards, letters and messages we've received?' I had absolutely no idea of the extent of what she was referring to. There were literally hundreds of letters of support and email messages and faxes from people all over the world. A lot of them I knew, of course—I had a wide network of friends, ex-playing mates and work associates. But what moved me more was the support from people I didn't know. To see their level of support really shook me. I decided that once I was out of hospital and recovering at my parents' house, I was going to reply to every single one of them. That mattered to me. After all, if someone I'd never met from Argentina or France or Canada was willing to write or type me a message of support, the very least I could do was reply. It would prove to be quite a job over the next few days, but it would form part of a routine that I was already composing in my head.

I'd previously asked Mum to bring in my laptop so that I could at least read some of my emails. Dad was already stressed about the number of visitors I was having, and he'd become worried that, by answering a few emails, I'd be doing too much.

I knew he hadn't been sleeping well because he was worried about me, but when he started being a bit negative about me doing anything, I had to say, 'Look Dad, me writing an email is like you writing a letter. It's not a difficult thing. It takes me thirty seconds.' I knew that he was tired and I knew that his desire to limit my activity was coming from a place of concern, but I didn't need negativity at that time. So I also said, 'The best thing you can do when you come in is be more upbeat. That's how *I'm* feeling at the moment and I want to keep it going.' He was much more positive and enthusiastic after that.

It was around that time too that I decided to get on Twitter. I'd always said that it would take a monumental event to initiate a tweet from me. I'd always been pretty cynical about Twitter and thought that it was self-serving and attention-seeking. I'd only ever used it as a news source.

So I decided that any tweet I put out would be purely informative. I got on my account and typed the words 'I'm still here.' That was it. It was direct and it said what I wanted it to. Anybody who'd heard what had happened and was wondering what the status was, well, here you go: 'I'm still here.' It's still there at the very bottom of my Twitter feed. I'm quite proud of it now. They were incredibly empowering words to type. Since then, I've viewed Twitter very differently. It remains a good news source, as it always has been, but I received, and still receive, lots of nice messages from people. I always try my best to reply to everyone, even if it's just a word or two. It would be a shame to not continue that communication.

SIXTEEN

SMALL GOALS; LITTLE MILESTONES

WHEN I WAS DISCHARGED from hospital, the feeling of euphoria was enormous. Dad came to pick me up, but before I left I went down to the ICU area to thank everyone who had been so good to me, and to say goodbye. Hospitals don't normally allow patients to do that, but they gave me a special dispensation, and I'm glad they did. Those nights when I was freezing cold or screaming in pain, these people were always there, trying to help me. I felt that we had bonded on some level. And it wasn't just me who needed help. There were ten or twelve other patients in ICU, also needing care.

All day, every day—these people keep doing the same things. Everyone I encountered in ICU was truly amazing, although, because of the shift roster, they weren't all in the ward the day I left. I just can't overstate how lucky I was to have been in that hospital in Brisbane. I had the right people around me at the right time, and without that the outcome could have been very different.

Now that I'd been discharged and was staying at my parents' house, I needed to deal with all the press attention. It was Brisbane; I was from Brisbane. The press were all over us. It felt like there was this thing needing to be fed, and that we had no choice but to feed it. They just wouldn't let go until we did. The day before I left hospital, I remember going over to the window of the ward and looking outside for the first time in more than a week. To my amazement, the car park in front of the hospital was full of TV crews from various networks, waiting to get some kind of comment. I remember thinking, 'We're going to have to handle this the right way.'

I'd left the hospital without speaking to the press and the question now was whether I should speak to all the newspapers and TV channels individually. That would take time and be exhausting. I didn't need that; nobody needed it. Of course there was the option not to talk at all, but I never seriously considered doing that.

While I was in hospital, a few of the rugby guys had taken on the role of fielding the enquiries that were coming in on my behalf. It was almost as if a makeshift Brisbane old-boys' network had swung into action. I'll never be able to repay those guys for what they did.

Slacky, with his vast experience as a producer at Brisbane's Channel 9 News, was probably at the top of the communication pyramid. Then below him you had other rugby guys like Timmy Horan and David Coe fielding phone calls from rugby connections all over the world. I couldn't possibly have spoken to everyone who called from the world of rugby—there were hundreds of ex-players calling, all hoping for news that I was okay.

Another friend who was very active in the communication was former Wallaby Mark Loane. Mark is a very able man in the field of ophthalmology—one of the best in Australia—and, when he heard about my stroke, not only was he very supportive but he also did a lot of helpful research into the visual aspects of my symptoms. Then you had my parents dealing with close family friends, and Isabella being the point of contact back in London. Others generously helped whenever they could. All these people acted as conduits for communication from people from different areas of my life. That was vital for me. It took the pressure off and spread the workload.

ANDREW SLACK: Michael's story was big news everywhere in Australia. He was very well known. With my experience of the media working at Channel 9 News, I knew for a fact that the best way to deal with the press would be to talk to them all at one single event, organised by us. You sit them down, answer all the questions they have and then they leave. By doing it that way, you essentially kill the story and they leave you alone thereafter. I strongly advised Michael and his father that this would be the best approach in this situation.

It had been a very tense period for Dad and a very concerning period for him. He always puts on a strong outward front, but I know that, inside, he feels things. Once I got out of the danger area and started recovering, I think that, because he had experience of brain issues and brain injuries, he was a bit shocked, as the doctors were, by the great improvement I was making every day, with no side effects other than the impaired vision.

So even when I was staying with Mum and Dad, he was still worrying all the time, urging me to slow down. He knew my personality and he was wary of me taking on too much too soon. It got to the point where I had to have a chat with him and say, 'Look Dad, I'm okay. I know where I stand. I almost understand what's going on.' I felt that I had an awareness of my own body's needs. I also told him about the rule I'd created for myself. 'If I'm tired, I sleep.' I still stick by that rule now.

Because of his career in psychology, Dad probably analyses people's behaviour more than the average person. He saw a difference in me, I think, and that seemed to concern him. Admittedly, I was talking a lot, but I *knew* I was talking a lot. I wasn't doing it because something about my brain was different. I was doing it because I was excited—'I've survived!' But I also knew that I had to temper that euphoria by making sure that I got enough rest. It was a balance I had to find.

MARIE LYNAGH: We saw him as being much more compulsive than previously. He was very talkative, compulsively talkative. Driven. He was also really enjoying his food and eating very quickly. In fact everything was done at pace. We asked Rob Henderson if it was possible there was some increased frontal lobe activity [the part of the brain that controls emotional reaction], but he didn't see it as being a factor.

For me, recovery was all about setting small, physically orientated goals. Little milestones. I'd done it in hospital with the trip to the bathroom, the walking, the exercises, the reading and watching TV. These were all measures for me. A means of gauging how my strength was returning and how I was adjusting to what was, for all intents and purposes, new eyesight. And I'd over-achieved on pretty much every one of those goals.

Staying at my parents' house in downtown Brisbane was a great way to recuperate. I'd been in regular contact with Isabella and the boys and I felt that they were carrying on with life, safe in the knowledge that I'd be home when the time was right. As much as I was receiving support in Australia from friends, Isabella was getting the same level of support at home: people offering to take the kids to school or sports commitments; families offering to have the kids to stay over to allow Isabella some time to rest. I knew this was taking a lot out of her, but it's not in her nature to complain. She just gets on with whatever she has to do to keep the family going, and that meant everything to me. The result was that I could focus totally on resting and getting better.

A few days after my discharge, we decided, on Slacky's advice, to hold a press conference back at the hospital. Slacky made sure that all the press were informed, and the theory was that they'd come along, listen to my announcement, ask a few questions and then it would all be over. I thought it was a great idea. Also, though I was tired, I wanted to test myself by seeing if I was capable of doing it. Dad wasn't so sure. He thought that I was pushing myself too hard.

Interestingly, a guy who wanted to do a special on me for a TV show in Australia called *Australian Story* also approached me shortly after leaving hospital. It's on the ABC and it's very good. As the name suggests, they do stories about Australians and they wanted to do one on me. At the time I said no. It was just too soon and I wasn't ready. He was very understanding and didn't push at all. I just wanted to focus on my recovery. Funnily enough, it turned out that his wife was one of the nurses in intensive care. I couldn't help but ask him, 'Well, how did I go?' At first he said, 'Oh, you were fine.' I went, 'I bet I wasn't!' and he said, 'Ah, well ...' I'm sure I wasn't the easiest. I don't think anyone's at his or her best in intensive care!

IAN LYNAGH: We were probably more cautious in managing him than he wanted us to be. I personally thought Michael was pushing himself too hard but, equally, I thought that it was probably the best approach. I knew the press would want their story. In the end I was amazed by what he was capable of doing. He wanted to walk in unaided and the press were amazed by how well he looked. It took a hell of a lot out of him, but he did it very professionally and courteously by thanking all the important people.

The press conference I gave at the hospital with Rob Henderson wasn't as big a deal for me as other people thought it was. I wasn't exactly enamoured with public speaking in general, but I'd obviously done it in the past. But it was emotional discussing what had happened with people outside family and close friends, even though I knew a good proportion of the people in the room because most of them were sports journalists. It wasn't as if I was batting on a tough wicket, either; they weren't there to ask me awkward questions like 'Why did Australia perform so poorly in the World Cup?' It was supportive: 'Good on you—thanks for coming out and talking to us' was the sentiment. I think I did it well and it was a good opportunity to publicly thank Rob and everyone who'd been so good to me. The first thing I said was, 'If you're going to have a stroke, have it here.' How very true that was.

SEVENTEEN

A STRANGER'S STORY

I WENT FOR A lot of long walks along the Brisbane River when I was recovering at my parents' house. They came with me for the first couple of weeks, as I was very tentative and was still adjusting to the changes in my vision. Though I could walk a fair distance without too much trouble, my balance was affected somewhat. Also, there were some safety issues. The path along the riverside didn't always have railings and there was a sheer drop to the river, fifteen feet below. It was dangerous, and the fact that the path was used by cyclists only made it more so. It took me a while to become familiar with the surroundings, now that I was viewing them through altered eyes. So initially I needed a bit of guidance to get my confidence back, though I was determined that that wasn't going to take very long.

The hardest part about the walking was getting to the river, which involved crossing a number of roads. I discovered that I could hear cars coming, but not bicycles, and it was eerie having to rely on senses other than my eyesight. But my mentality was pretty much as it had been throughout: I needed to understand what I was capable of. I needed to establish a baseline of ability to build from—'Okay, today I can do this. What can I do tomorrow?'

When Mum and Dad were confident that I was able to venture out on my own, I pushed myself a little further. I'd probably been out of hospital for two weeks. It felt like I was a child again—'I'll be back around 3pm!' When I got back from walking each day, I'd lie down and sleep for four hours or more. It was deep, dark sleep—not unlike that night in the hospital when my recovery began. I needed it.

IAN LYNAGH: He was incredibly driven about his desire to walk. He was crossing major streets in Brisbane and he was determined to do it on his own. I used to basically hold my breath for three hours every time he left the house. We'd peer out the window, waiting for him to come round the corner. It was always a relief— 'He's coming! He's coming!' He was incredibly strongly self-managed.

When I wasn't sleeping or walking, I read a lot and answered the hundreds of emails and letters that had been sent to me. Every single one of them received a response of some kind when the return address was available to me. It was emotional reading them all and hearing from people I hadn't heard from for years. What surprised me was that while I got a huge amount of correspondence from players of my era and later, there were also lots of letters and emails from people who'd played the game long before me. I hadn't met most of them, but it meant everything to me that they cared enough to get in touch.

IAN LYNAGH: Michael had a formal routine for the whole time he was staying with us. Typical of ex-sportsmen, his recovery focus was very much on the physical, as opposed to the emotional. Every day was an exercise in making one more forward step in terms of his physical wellbeing, but he wasn't really open to discussing anything else. That's pretty typical of him. Any time we asked him how he was, which we did pretty regularly, he'd just say, 'All's well', and carry on with his routine.

I GUESS, IN RETROSPECT, my way of addressing everything that had happened was to focus on my physical capabilities. I'd go to the practice putting green at Royal Queensland Golf Club with Dad to see how my putting was affected by my reduced vision. I'd take that idea further by hitting a few chips, hitting a few easy 6-iron shots on the practice range and then attempting to play a hole of golf. It was all part of testing myself in a physical sense in environments that I liked and that were important to me.

IAN LYNAGH: I don't think the intrinsic value of golf itself was important to Michael. I think it was more a case of him proving to himself that he was alive and well by doing something that (a) he enjoyed and (b) he associated with when he was healthy. I wasn't happy with him doing it, but it's Michael we're talking about.

As much as I was focused on my physical recovery, I was also aware of the emotional rollercoaster a stroke puts you through. I'd read that mood swings and depression were part of the process and I was mindful of accepting these emotions and dealing with them in the best way I could. That said, emotions had never been something I was particularly comfortable discussing, prior to the stroke—not unlike most men, I suspect. Now I knew I'd have to devote as much attention to them as to my physical wellbeing. I suppose I felt that the attention I was giving the physical symptoms could only help the emotional ones, and I still believe that. What is it they say? 'Fit mind, fit body.'

One day changed my views slightly, however. It was a bright Tuesday; perfect weather. Not a cloud in the sky; warm, but not hot. As I left my parents' house I felt glad to be alive for all sorts of reasons. The euphoria of having survived was tangible and the feeling that I had been relatively spared was very strong. It came over me in a rush of happiness, as it did most days.

I was due to meet Mick (the guy who'd brought me the chewing gum and surfing magazines in hospital) for a coffee at Southbank—a public facility that comprises art galleries, the State Library, cafes, restaurants and even a beach and swimming area complete with lifeguards—right in the middle of the city. Mick's office was nearby.

It was only about an hour's walk from my parents' inner-city house to the cafe. Mick and I were chatting about nothing in particular when I noticed a man arrive on a tricycle. It seemed to be a modified bike; it was about the same size except with three wheels. I noticed that the man was helped as he dismounted and made his way to a nearby table. I didn't think much about it and continued with our chat.

About ten minutes later the guy approached our table. He walked awkwardly and very slowly. He said hello. He sounded drunk, but he clearly wasn't. Then he said, 'I just wanted to say how pleased I am to see you well and recovering.' He held out his right hand and I shook it in thanks. I could feel that his hand had very little power. He struggled to even lift it. I asked him to join us.

His story was to change me significantly.

He'd had a stroke while driving his car. He then crashed his car into a light post as a result of losing consciousness. So not only did he have to deal with the injuries resulting from a serious car crash, but the stroke left him unable to talk or walk. He also lost the use of his right hand. His sight was badly affected. His life was altered beyond repair.

This young man had been in his final year of medical studies and had been engaged to be married. He could not complete his studies and his fiancée left him, unable to deal with his physical deterioration. He told me that he'd had to move from Adelaide, where he lived, to Brisbane. He had no family and Brisbane offered the only facility where he could be cared for and recover.

For some reason our paths crossed that day. I've often wondered why. He was out on his daily ride on his tricycle with his physiotherapist and I was having my daily walk, meeting my friend. Two strangers with something in common. It was a totally random event, but an extremely powerful one. Because of a stroke, this young man's life had taken a devastating turn for the worse.

When he left us, I was very upset. I cried. It was as if this meeting had opened a compartment in me that I'd been desperately trying to keep tightly closed. It was the place where my emotions were stored. I just couldn't fathom how his life could have been so drastically impacted by a stroke, whereas

I'd suffered the same thing and was relatively okay. Why was I spared and he wasn't? I'd attended a Catholic school as a child, but I'd never been a particularly religious man. I thought, 'Who decides?'

I was getting into deeply emotional territory. I obviously hadn't reconciled what had happened to me. I hadn't had the opportunity. All I felt at that moment was guilt that it wasn't me on the tricycle—'Why was this guy's life torn apart and not mine?' I couldn't make sense of any of it. I regret not taking the guy's name. I went back later to the Southbank cafe to see if I could find him, but I never managed to. I enquired if anyone knew of his whereabouts but got no leads.

Mick was very moved by what he saw in me. But he's also a pretty knockabout guy who doesn't mince his words. He looked at me and said, 'Mate, you should not feel guilty. You are lucky—extremely lucky. What you need to do is use that luck to help others.'

He was absolutely correct. I *was* very lucky.

When I started to weigh it all up, it occurred to me how truly lucky I'd been in so many ways. I'd been lucky in terms of how little damage I'd been left with. That was the obvious first thought. In a broader sense I started thinking about how fortunate I'd been to have had the stroke in Brisbane, where a lot of people knew who I was. I had my parents, great medical staff who could see me quickly, and great friends who had the presence of mind to get me to hospital.

Not just that—once I was in hospital, I had several great networks of friends looking out for me, visiting me, communicating with hundreds of well-wishers from all over the world on my behalf. And as if that wasn't enough, *another* network of fantastic people had thought nothing of dropping everything to help Isabella and the boys back at home. Who gets that kind of good fortune? I got it—it really was amazing.

Equally, I couldn't help thinking how differently everything could have turned out. What if I'd had the stroke in the hotel in Singapore before I even got to Brisbane? I could have had a headache at dinner and gone up to my room. Then what? I would have been in serious trouble. I'd have been in a strange city, miles from people who knew me

Worse still, imagine if I'd had the stroke on a flight? Then what do you do? The possible outcome there isn't even worth considering. I definitely don't think I'd be here, writing this book.

SO, HAVING ANALYSED HOW very lucky I was in every conceivable respect, from that moment on I set my mind to finding a way to help people who hadn't walked away from a stroke as well as I had. I didn't know what that formula would be at that point, but I knew that if I continued to think about it, something would evolve in the months ahead.

It wasn't the last time I'd feel pangs of guilt, of course. I think that's a process that everyone who survives a stroke goes through. You go with it, acknowledge the emotions you feel and try to find a way to channel them positively rather than letting the guilt consume you. Yes, I wanted to help people— that's great. But how was I going to actually do it? The answers would come to me in time.

EIGHTEEN

REUNION

THERE ARE A FEW questions you ask yourself in the aftermath of a stroke. One of them for me was: 'Why did my artery split the way it did?'

It was a question that I asked myself many times in the quiet hours when I was staying at Mum and Dad's. I still wonder sometimes. People might assume that a career playing contact sport must have weakened something and led to a situation where the artery was prone to dissection. But I've been told that's not likely. What's more probable is that my artery rupture was caused by a perfect storm of circumstances.

There'll never be a cut-and-dried answer and it's probably easier to move forward that way. I'd stopped playing in 1998 and the doctors felt that if rugby had contributed to the traumatic event of stroke there would have been symptoms at that time.

I've learned that neurologists are a practically minded bunch. They focus on what's actually presented in the scans on the day they are taken. They won't speculate on what may or may not have been happening in the background, because it just doesn't matter. Neurologists deal in fact, in reality, and in those terms all that mattered was that my artery split. Their concern was how to limit the damage.

As I've said, the cause was likely to have been a combination of a few seemingly more mundane factors. I was sleep-deprived, jetlagged, probably dehydrated, and had been vigorously swinging a golf club. All these factors—topped off by that single unforeseeably traumatic moment when I choked and coughed on the beer—were probably enough to cause the artery to split. I couldn't have predicted it and certainly couldn't have protected myself against it. It was simply one of those events that blindsides you. All you can do is hope you survive to tell the story. Hope it's not your turn to go.

But I couldn't help recalling a few episodes I'd experienced in the year or so prior to the stroke. 'What was all that about?' I wondered.

I can only describe them as dizzy turns, and they only happened occasionally. Whenever they did, I'd be puzzled as to the cause, although I don't think I was ever concerned enough to mention it to Isabella. I thought, 'I'll be fine,' never, 'Oh hell, here comes a stroke.'

Commonly, it would happen when I stood up after I'd been lying down for a while. The room would spin for a few seconds and it would take me a few more to get my orientation again. Sometimes, when I was lying down in bed, the room would spin as if I'd had too much to drink. It was a strange sensation. But then it would go away.

I just put it down to my stressful lifestyle: long hours at work, not enough sleep, maybe—it was nothing to get worried about and certainly not worth a trip to the doctor. But I do remember asking Rob Henderson in our initial conversations if there was any likely connection to the artery splitting. 'Was that a warning?' I was aware of the concept of the mini-stroke: a minor stroke, or series of strokes, that can be almost unnoticeable. They can happen to anyone at any age and are often considered a precursor to something major.

Rob's response was that he couldn't even begin to consider whether these incidents were related to the stroke. The absence of scan images prior to the stroke made speculation pointless. There may have been a slight defect, but, equally, there may not have been. It's just impossible to tell after the event.

ISABELLA LYNAGH: Michael never mentioned any serious prior health issues to me, because if he had, I would have been the first person to suggest that he should go and see a doctor. In the months prior to the stroke, however, I did notice that he was very stressed and prone to outbursts of anger and frustration, and I remember thinking that something bad could happen during one of these because of the inevitable rise in blood pressure. That's the only thought I ever had. Michael can take things pretty seriously sometimes and can get worked up about things that I don't necessarily think are important. As a result, he'd get himself in a bit of a mental 'hole' of negativity quite easily when he felt something was going against him.

Any time I went back to Royal Brisbane Hospital for a follow-up scan, I'd take the opportunity to quiz Rob Henderson on the specifics of what had happened in my head. To his credit, he always had time for me. I wasn't his only patient and he'd dealt with hundreds of cases like mine. I just needed to understand as much as I possibly could. And, three years later, there are still aspects of the stroke that I'm not completely clear about. I still email Rob now and again with questions—'So what exactly is that white area I'm seeing in the scan image?'

Initially I just wanted to know what the prognosis for my vision was. Was this it? Was I always going to be missing the left side of my field of vision? Would it improve? Could it get worse?

Rob had no definitive answers for that and the reason he didn't is that there aren't any. Generally speaking, damage caused by a stroke that affects the occipital lobe—the part of the brain that controls vision—is not reversible. That said, some people in my situation have experienced improvements over time. For the first few weeks I used to close my eyes at night, hoping that I'd wake up in the morning to find my sight had improved. Sometimes I'd think it actually had. When I asked Rob about it, he was always circumspect, and that I understand.

When you think about it, your brain has to go through a complex series of adjustments following a stroke. That won't happen overnight. But gradually, the brain will find a way to compensate for impaired vision, for example. Your eyesight might not be any better, but it might *seem* to be better because of the compensation going on. Even that is good. I'll take that.

During one of the many follow-up scans I had after I'd left hospital, we were very concerned to be told that there was a tiny area of new stroke showing up on the images. It hadn't caused any new symptoms and it was located in an area on the other side of the back of my brain called the right visual cortex. I certainly had not been aware of any pain or discomfort that might have indicated something new happening.

DR HENDERSON: We do it [follow-up scans] to establish the safety of the artery, and Michael had a few more scans than most people get because of his medical history. Also, we didn't exactly expect him to be out playing golf so soon after. But one scan showed a tiny, new area of stroke. I showed Michael's pictures to quite a few well-known neurologists down in Melbourne who were following his progress with interest. All the new scan made us do was change his medication from using aspirin to clopidigrel—an oral anti-platelet agent used to inhibit blood clots. When I showed another guy the scan he said, 'If you scan anyone within a two-week period, you'll probably always find a couple of little tiny strokes.' He [Michael] wouldn't have noticed anything; it was just a tiny dot on the scan to keep people on their toes. This was the second-last scan before he could fly, given that we normally like to allow a month from a stroke from a flying viewpoint.

Because I couldn't fly for a certain period after my stroke, I ended up being in Australia much longer than I'd intended. Originally I was to be there for three days, but it ended up being six weeks. Rather than waiting any longer, Isabella and I decided it would be great if she came out to visit me. She arranged for one of our many helpful friends back home to look after the kids for ten days or so.

When she arrived in mid-May, it was an incredibly emotional reunion. We hugged and we just couldn't let go; she commented on how skinny I was. 'I thought I'd lost you,' she said. I think that was one of the moments when I realised just what we'd all been through. She was clearly exhausted, as I was, but to be back together seemed to give me renewed energy.

ISABELLA LYNAGH: When Michael met me at the airport, I couldn't believe how much weight he'd lost. I just could not let go of him. We've never been a very publicly affectionate couple. We don't kiss and hold hands in public all the time, but during the ten days we spent together in Brisbane, I don't think I ever let his hand go. The whole event made us both realise how important life is and we've been a lot more affectionate ever since.

On one of her first days in Brisbane, I had a scan scheduled at the hospital. After the previous slightly worrying one, when the new speck of stroke damage showing on the scan had given us a few tense moments, it was vital to my hopes of flying home that my scan was indicative of stability.

We went in, I had the scan and then sat in the office waiting for the results while Isabella waited a little nervously in the corridor. Then one of the nurses came in and said, 'Wait here, the doctors want to see you.' I was thinking to myself, 'This can't be good. If everything was fine, surely they'd just tell me.' Five minutes later, Rob Henderson came into the office and said, 'Everything's fine.' It was a great moment. We sat there chatting for what turned into forty minutes and finally he said, 'Shouldn't you go and tell your wife?' I said, 'Oh my God, yes!'

I went out and told Isabella the good news. She'd been sitting there worried. As we left and were saying goodbye to Rob, he said to Isabella, 'Now go and buy your husband a very nice glass of wine.' We went home, got dressed up and went out for a beautiful dinner with my parents. It was a significant step in the right direction.

A couple of days later we decided that we wanted to get away for a bit, so we booked into a hotel in Noosa, a beautiful beach resort up the coast from Brisbane. I thought it would be a nice change of scene for me. It sounds ridiculous but I was actually wary of telling my parents what we were planning because I knew they'd disapprove, thinking I was overdoing it. In the end, I explained to them that I'd just be sitting in the passenger seat while Isabella drove the rental car for the ninety-minute journey to Noosa. I said, 'It's no more strenuous than sitting in the house. I'll be fine.' After a little more reassuring they were okay about it so Isabella and I took off and spent a few days relaxing in Noosa Heads.

It was the first time since leaving hospital that I'd had a proper chance to decompress. We walked on the beach every day, had nice meals. It was here that I really started to realise how great it was to be alive. I'd battled to improve my physical abilities and tested myself every day for weeks in all manner of disciplines. I'd walked; I'd tested my sight in every way I could. Now I just needed time to reflect and to relax with Isabella. It occurred to me that everything was going to turn out well.

The night before I flew back home to London, I asked the guys who'd been with me in Friday's on the night of the stroke if they wanted to go out again. I said, 'Guys, we're going to finish this. And do it in a better way than last time.' Last time I went out for a beer, I ended up in hospital for almost two weeks. I needed closure of some kind. I also needed that whole sequence of my life to end on a positive note.

They agreed, and when we met at Friday's I said, 'This time I actually want to get through it', and with that I took a sip from a little seven-ounce beer. For me it felt good and, more

NINETEEN

BACK TO WORK

AFTER I GOT BACK from Australia and all the euphoric 'I'm home! Wasn't it great that we beat it!' stuff had died down, there came a moment when I had to accept that life simply goes on. Everybody was really happy to see me—of course they were—but then, one day, it felt as if they were looking at me and thinking, 'He's over it now. There's nothing wrong with him. Life goes on.'

To a certain extent, that was true. I know that. But one of the things I found, and still find, frustrating about my situation is that to look at me nobody would even know that I'd had a stroke. I look the same; I sound the same. You wouldn't know. But *I* know. I had a stroke and my vision is impaired as a result. I had a stroke when my artery split and my brain became swollen. It happened. Life has changed for me. I don't see like I used to. I can no longer drive a car. That's not easy after thirty years, especially with three young boys needing to be ferried around at weekends. There are also a lot of other things that are affected: golf, riding a bike, surfing—all pastimes that are important to me.

So sometimes I wish I could wear a sign around my neck—'Stroke victim! I can't see very well!'—for all the people who get pissed off when I accidentally bump into them on the Underground. I actually get a fright myself because I genuinely don't see people coming. Despite that, I get the impression that there are some members of the general public, even some friends, who when they meet me think, 'Well, what was all the fuss about? Look at him. There's nothing wrong with him. It must have been a really minor stroke.'

Certainly when I first came home I really did get the feeling that some people thought I'd made a bit of a fuss about nothing. Built it up much bigger than what it was. I certainly hadn't. It was never my intention to be even remotely public about what had happened. At the time when the story was in the papers and on TV I thought: 'It must be a really slow news week if I'm in the front pages.'

I talked about the stroke and recovery a lot during that first month back home. People wanted to know. We'd have friends round for dinner and the first question was always, 'So, tell us what happened ...'

I'd tell them the story in a fair bit of detail, to the point where I actually got pretty good at telling it. A little bit of humour here and there and you brush it off. It's easier to see the humorous side of situations when you've survived them.

But when I talked about the incredible people I'd met, the neurologists, the nurses, the guy who cleans the blood off the ward floor every day, people were eerily quiet. I'd say, 'What's wrong?' And they always said, 'Don't you mind talking about this stuff?' I'd say, 'Not at all!' Part of me needed to talk about it, to remind me of what I'd survived.

But I always said to Isabella, 'If I ever start going on too long about this and people are getting bored, please tell me.' You know what it's like when people talk far too much about anything.

Take skiing, for example. Don't get me wrong, skiing's nice—I like skiing. But I don't want to hear about it for hours on end. I don't think anybody does. When I go surfing, I'm pretty sure I don't come home and go, 'Well, the surf was this and this and this …' I prefer to keep it brief. Someone asks, 'How was the surfing?' I'll just say something like, 'Yeah, we had a few good days', or 'There was no surf', unless they ask more. Then I'll happily bore them for days …

So I was very aware of not boring people with my story, though generally people seemed very interested. A lot of them were my age or even a bit younger, so I'm sure a few were thinking, 'This could happen to me.'

But the hardest part of recovery was the coming down from euphoria to deal with the more mundane moments of life. Once you come down, there's that risk that you keep going down. I definitely understand how people end up getting depressed. I've been there, not too badly, but enough to recognise it and to know that the abyss is there and waiting.

Whenever I felt myself sliding, I said to myself, 'Don't even go there, mate. Get out of this.' That's my personality. It's the same trait that, with five minutes to go in a rugby match when you need a try to win, makes you say to yourself, 'I'm going to find a way to win this—to turn this situation around', not, 'Oh, well we can't win this. We're out of the World Cup.' Despite that, I've still had more than a few moments where things have got pretty heavy and I've thought to myself, 'I'm not sure if I can get out of this.'

It's usually family motivations that have hauled me out of the emotional depths. Looking after the kids, seeing them grow up and enjoying my role as a father, husband and financial provider. I think I hold these roles even more dearly now than I did before the stroke.

Previously, I might too easily have got caught up in the stresses of life. I think I'm a lot calmer now and I definitely appreciate how much Isabella does for the family. It's funny, when I first came home I told her, 'Look, I need to rest as much as possible. So it might be that I need to lie down on the couch most afternoons and sleep.' She didn't even blink. She said, 'Nothing's changed, then. You used to do that before you had a stroke!'

I joke, but I do recognise that life has become tougher for her. Because I can't drive, and because I used to do a good share of driving the kids around, that's put a lot of extra pressure on her. But like I said, she never complains. She does whatever is needed and I often wonder how much all of this has taken out of her. I wish I could discuss it more but I genuinely don't find that kind of conversation easy. That's a weakness of mine, I know that, and it's something I'm committed to work on. Life really is too short not to talk openly with the people you love.

ISABELLA LYNAGH: Michael has been more affectionate and definitely more grateful [since the stroke]. Overall, I know that he's definitely more aware of his mortality and I think he's trying hard to control his moods. He's definitely more aware of how fragile life is and the fact that he can't see properly must be a constant reminder. In terms of how it has all affected me, it has been a strain. Michael has always worked, so he wasn't always there to help anyway.

But it is a big strain at the weekends. I have adapted, but I am still suffering. I was so strong for the weeks when Michael was at his lowest, then you realise that you've just got nothing left. I still worry about him and all that stress does have physical manifestations for me. I feel like I have post-traumatic stress sometimes. It has to come out somehow. I don't really talk about these problems with Michael, though. It's not that he doesn't recognise what I'm dealing with, because he does. It's more a case of everyday life taking over.

For the kids there were adjustments to make. They all seem to have responded very well, although Isabella always says that Thomas, our middle son, felt it most. He's definitely the most sensitive of the three.

When I first came home, I made a point of explaining to them, in simple terms, what had happened. But they are kids; it's asking a lot to expect them to really understand it all. In the end we just reminded them, 'Daddy can't see very well on his left side, so be careful how you approach him and what you leave lying around the floor.' I think they all understood. They even managed to trick me a few times by doing things in the part of my vision that they knew was affected. Sometimes they still do it. Making light of the situation seems to make it easier.

Seeing fellow stroke survivors has been another huge leveller for me, especially in those moments when I've been close to feeling, 'Why me?' I've been approached by a number of organisations that deal with stroke in some way, in both the UK and Australia. Isabella and I were invited to the Life After Stroke awards lunch in London in 2012, organised by the Stroke Association. It was my first public appearance since the stroke. It was pretty daunting to be around crowds of people. I'd been in contact with the people at the Stroke Association on and off and they wanted me to present an award. The event recognises achievements by people who have survived a stroke and those who give care: volunteers, medical professionals and carers. It's a cry-athon—there's no other way of describing it. It's very emotional. There were two hundred people in the audience and everybody was crying—it was an outpouring of emotion for people who have managed to keep their lives going despite serious disability.

That day made me view things differently. And it took me one step further down the road that leads away from survivor's guilt. Part of me, looking at badly afflicted survivors of stroke, still thinks, 'That could have been me.' That might always be the case; we'll see. But there's a much bigger part of me that now thinks, 'I had this upside down. I'm not giving to them; they are giving to me.'

At the lunch I sat next to a young man who'd had a stroke while heading a football. He was in his mid to late thirties, perhaps; he was from Jersey. When he'd gone up to head the ball, his head had collided with his opponent's head. Initially, he merely felt dizzy, maybe a little concussed, but then he went home and had a full-blown stroke. His speech isn't great, he can't write; he's a youngish guy with a wife and children. He was a writer, and now he has to use his iPad to communicate by typing answers to questions and showing you the screen. He told me that, despite his disabilities, he'd recently run the Jersey marathon in some incredibly long time. That part didn't matter; it was the fact that he'd finished that meant everything.

When I hear these people's stories, I find them incredibly powerful. My pulse quickens when they talk about what they've been through. For those few moments I almost forget I've been through a similar thing. It's inspirational to see perfectly normal people who've been struck down—their lives changed to the point where they don't want to go on—turn it around, saying, 'No, I still have a life. It might not be the one I planned before the stroke, but at least I have it. Many others don't.'

It takes a certain type of human being to say that.

By showing how they can overcome disability and keep going, these people are actually giving to 'normal' people by saying, 'Hey, look what I've made of my situation. You think you've got it tough?' They don't actually say that, of course; they just get on with it. I think it's magnificent. If I could do that, that would make me feel fulfilled.

As I've mentioned, my problem is that people see me and say, 'You're all right.' I sometimes wish I could tell them more about what I've been through, what I'm still going through. I sometimes feel like saying, 'Spend a day in my shoes'—not that I would wish that on anybody. Because I look 'normal' and act 'normal', there's this, 'Michael's okay, on to the next one' attitude. That's fair, because there are people who need care, assistance and attention an awful lot more than I do.

But I'm still a stroke survivor. I still feel I have something to offer in these discussions. I have a deep understanding of what these people have been through and huge admiration for what they've achieved. I can tell the story too; I can talk to them, sympathise with them and treat them as the people they are.

One guy, while giving a speech about his stroke, described the feeling of its onset as like getting hit on the back of the head with a baseball bat. I said, 'That's it. It's just how you describe it!' I used to call it a severe, sudden headache. But it wasn't just a headache; it was something much more. I thought, 'I'm going to use that from now on.' It's a great description, because everybody can relate to it.

The Stroke Association lunch reminded me, 'Jeez, you've been through a serious event. But you've come through it.' Every now and then I need reminding of that. It gives me strength. It's not that I'm bullet-proof; I was just very lucky in terms of where I was, the people I was with and the fact that I wasn't touched as badly as I could have been. The nature of Life After Stroke events is that you tend to meet people who really need medical services, support and care on a daily basis, whereas somebody like me doesn't need that.

There are also many people out there with my level of stroke damage. I've met a couple of people who have hemiopia, like I do. I was sitting in the eye doctor's office one day and the guy opposite me said, 'I have exactly what you have. It's great to meet you.' He had hemiopia on the opposite side. Mine is on the left side; his was on the right. We both actually said, 'We should go and watch a game of rugby together. We'd cover the whole field between us. You take one side, I'll cover the other. Then we'll be good!' I'm still in touch with that bloke.

I hope that because I'm someone who is, to some degree, in the public eye, I can be an inspiration to others. I don't hold myself out as any kind of shining light, far from it, but I support stroke-related research and raise money for it and stroke services, without making any kind of fanfare at all. I'm sure there are hundreds of people in the same boat. I just hope that if I talk to the people I meet about stroke and provide a little support, then because I have a bit of a profile, maybe people who didn't know much about stroke might learn something.

Previously I was one of those people who thought, 'Stroke is something that happens to old people.' I know for a fact that Isabella thought the same. Well, it's not. Stroke does not discriminate at all. Of course, if you're unfit and you smoke and drink, then yes, you're more likely to have one. But stroke can affect young kids too. It can even affect babies. It's a much bigger issue in our society than most people realise. If I can make people more aware of it, that's great.

Recognising the symptoms is really important too. Recognising that 'Let's not mess around with this; let's get to a doctor' type of moment, even if it turns out to be a false alarm, can be vital to survival and recovery. It's always better to be on the safe side, as I was—'Yes, you'd better call an ambulance.'

Meeting so many inspirational people at the Life After Stroke awards coincided with a conversation I had with James Gemmell, one of my colleagues at Sky. He had a family connection to stroke back in New Zealand and we were chatting while we were on air one Saturday. He said, 'Look, I'm thinking of running the London Marathon this year and I'd like to do it for the Stroke Association. Would you like to help?' I said, 'You know what, I think I might just run the marathon with you.' He said, '*Really?*' And I said, 'Yes.'

Then we came up with the idea of having something *specific* to raise money for, albeit under the umbrella of the Stroke Foundation. From previous experience—when I raised money for an athletics track for Stoke Mandeville in 2000—I knew that it helped to have a tangible focus.

Back then I'd said to Nigel Wray and Nick Leslau, 'Come on, let's run a marathon.' Nigel had run marathons before. Even Nick—a big guy who never had—said, 'Okay, I'll do it too.' The three of us raised £300,000, and a track was built for wheelchair- bound athletes. It was tangible. People could look at it and say, 'That's what my money went towards.'

In this instance, if we were to say, 'I'm raising money for the Stroke Association', people who get hit on by charities all the time would think, 'Oh, just another charity ...' So there had to be a special, meaningful, tangible goal to aim for so that people could say, 'Okay, *that's* where the money's going.' It's all about goals. Small steps.

And so that's how the Back to Work project was born and launched. The Stroke Association found other sponsors who, between them, agreed to match whatever we raised—the Association needed £300,000 to get the project off the ground. Sky got involved too and we had a Team Sky who agreed to run the marathon and raise money with James and me. Of particular significance to me personally was that the marathon was almost a year to the day since my stroke.

Why did I do it? I've often asked myself that. Part of it was my desire to continue to find a degree of physical closure for myself post-stroke, in combination with my inbuilt competitive nature. People said, 'But you've recovered well.' That was true. But I wanted a great recovery, and to run a marathon a year later qualified as great in my eyes.

Not that I actually ran it all. I didn't do a huge amount of running training; I did a lot of walking. My calves really blew up, probably while trying to protect my already bad knees, and so I said to myself, 'In the worst-case scenario, I'll walk the whole bloody thing!' I just wanted to finish it. That was my goal. I didn't want this 'I'm going to do a sub-four or a sub-three and a half' pressure. People would ask me what time I was aiming for and I'd tell them that my goal was to finish on the same day I started.

I'd never walked a marathon before. The first one that I ran took me four and a half hours, so heaven knows how long it would take to walk one. I tried to calculate it walking round Richmond Park. I'd talk to myself, saying things like, 'Well, if three laps equals X, it'll take so many hours to do this ...' I worked out that it would take me seven and a half hours to walk the marathon course. I thought, 'Well that's not toooo bad. It'll still be daylight ...'

When it came to it, I managed to run the first half before my calves completely gave in. I walked the last part, but I was in absolute agony. Interestingly, James Gemmell—who's light, fit and does a lot of running—had all kinds of problems. He'd trained really hard, was really keen and was going for a specific time.

But his calves blew out and I think his hamstring also went. Then he said, 'I don't think I can do it.' I felt really sorry for him; he was really disappointed. So I said, 'Mate ... just walk with me. We'll have a chat; we'll get round.' And that's exactly what we did. We walked it and we were still passing people at the end—people who were trying to run! I think it took us five and a half hours. James was great, as were all the people from Team Sky. It was an uplifting day.

We raised enough money to create the Back to Work project and make it an ongoing program for three years. Employees' salaries would be guaranteed for that period by the money we raised. The program is designed to help people back into the community. People always assume that when someone leaves hospital they're cured. Actually, that's just the start. Leaving hospital merely means that you've survived, and it's when you get home that the real issues start. That's when people need answers to questions like, 'What do I do? What am I *capable* of doing?'

Lots of people can't work as they used to after a stroke, so the Back to Work program aims to give people a reason to get out of bed in the morning—to do *something*, even if it isn't what they did before. It's really important to help people feel they are contributing, and to give them a sense of self-worth. It's a big thing and I'm really passionate about it. When it came to getting me back to work, I'd been lucky. The companies I was working for, as well as Sky, were very supportive and gave me time. Also, I'd remained very capable. But that's not always the case.

I remember my first day back at Sky after the stroke. I was to comment on the Australia v Wales Test. Gus Williamson, the head of rugby at Sky, said, 'You don't have to rush back to do this.' And I thought, 'Well, I'll be watching at home anyway.' If I worked I'd be driven to the studio, I'd sit there with people I know, talking about something I know, then I'd be driven home. It would all be over in two and a half hours. I thought, 'I can do that!' So I did and Sky were great.

They never put any pressure on me. It was more a case of my saying, 'Right, I'm ready.' There wasn't much of a downside for me, and that first call after the stroke worked okay. It was a big step and I do admit that I was a little apprehensive. As I've said, the smaller the screen, the easier it is for me. Once you get these big, wide screens, like the ones at Sky, I can't see the left-hand side of the screen.

So sometimes I'd be watching the ball carrier and all of a sudden a tackler would appear from the left and I'd say, 'God, where did he come from?' Fitzy would say, 'He was standing there, Michael!' I'm used to it now, but initially it was quite a shock.

By way of comparison, I heard one story about a young lady who was an accountant in a company. She had a stroke and the company was very supportive of her and said, 'When you're ready, back you come.' But she couldn't operate at the level she wanted to, or was used to. So, while the company was good to her, she said, 'I can't do this.'

They ended up finding her a role as a front-desk greeter, more or less. While much less senior than her previous job, to her it was important that she got up in the morning, got dressed and went to work. She had a meaningful role that she enjoyed and fitted her altered capabilities at her company, and without that she wouldn't have known what to do. That's what Back to Work is all about.

The program not only helps with jobs, CVs and training, it also helps with families. That's part of the whole Stroke Association remit. It's not just the survivors they help; it's the people around them, who are often forgotten. I know that in my family Isabella has to do things—simple things—that I can't. That's really tough on her, and it's tough on me too because I miss taking the kids to parties or sports at the weekend. But in some cases people need full-time carers, or have to adapt their housing situation because they can't walk up stairs. It's really stressful on everybody involved and often it's the families who are forgotten.

TWENTY
THE PUNDIT

PEOPLE, INCLUDING EX-PLAYERS AND colleagues, often ask me, 'How did you get into doing all the media stuff?'

I certainly never set out to become a pundit. But I never did anything to burn that bridge while I was still playing either. When people asked me questions after games, or Sky or anyone else did special pieces with me for shows like *The Rugby Club*, because I had a wide range of interests outside rugby, my pieces tended to be interesting and a little insightful. An anecdote here, a funny quote there—something to show that I'd given the question a bit of thought rather than saying the first thing that came into my head.

I didn't do this because I wanted a job in broadcasting. I did it because that's how I am. I've always tried to develop a broad palette of interests. I think that it dates back to the amateur days of rugby, when your closest teammates might be a lawyer, a farmer and a doctor. You can't help but absorb some of that knowledge. I always encourage people to learn as much as possible about areas that aren't part of their daily life. That's also the advice I give young guys now when they say, 'I want to get into broadcasting.' It's even more pertinent in the professional game to try to broaden your horizons because just about everyone a player interacts with is another rugby professional.

I always think that when you get a chance to get in front of the camera or know you're going to be interviewed after a game, you should do some preparation. That's your shop window. Give it thought. Try and be entertaining. Don't just roll out the clichés like 'Hats off to the opposition' or 'It's a game of two halves', which everybody just tunes out. Say something interesting. You don't have to be controversial. Just be analytically astute. Use words that other people don't use. There's no need to give away team secrets or criticise people. Just say something that people might not know.

Lawrence Dallaglio used to be really good at it when he was playing. He was a captain and a big character, so he was often interviewed. Even so, he'd always have an interesting way of presenting something new. He'd have a little quote that you'd guess he'd probably rehearsed, but he'd bang it out and it was always good television. No wonder he's done very well and is in big demand.

A slightly different example is Nick Cummins—the 'Honey Badger'. That persona has taken on a life of its own. He's got the Australian rhyming slang, he's knockabout, he laughs, he has a bit of fun. Sky can't get enough of him. That's his style. 'Good on you,' I think when he comes on.

Don't get me wrong, I don't want twenty of him, but if you get the chance, as he does, say something interesting.

Being interesting in interviews paid dividends for me, because, just before I retired in 1998, Sky asked me to come along and be one of the guest analysts for a game—I can't remember which one. The reason they did that was, yes, because I was a well-known player, fresh out of the game, but also because I'd always tried to be insightful in interviews, some of them with Sky. For them, that was an attractive combination.

At first it went like this. Sky would ring and say, 'Can you come and do this game?'

'Okay, sure. That'd be good,' I'd say.

Then it was, 'How about this one too, and the next one?'

'No problem.'

And on it went. They kept asking and I kept going. First there was no contract—it was an informal week-to-week arrangement. Then it was a one-year deal and finally a two-year rolling contract. It's been that way ever since. We just sit down and they say, 'Do you want to keep doing this?' And I say, 'Yes.'

Technically speaking I'm not employed by Sky; I'm a contracted 'talent'. I like the game. I enjoy watching it and I think I have some good things to say—things to enhance the action and add a bit of colour to what's patently obvious. I've covered all the premiership games for Sky. There've been some great games when I've thought, 'I love this', and there've been others when it's January, freezing cold and it's 0–0 at halftime. On those days I'd think, 'Is this what I really want to be doing today?' But life's like that. You make the best of what's in front of you. It's rugby—there's *something* to comment on in every game.

The key is to steer clear of the inane stuff, but sometimes it's unavoidable. Sometimes during the show you'll get thrown a question that you're not prepared for or have no answer for—or you've only got ten seconds to answer it. Then you'll come up with one of those 'Well, whoever scores first … will score first' or 'Whoever scores first will have an advantage' type of statements. I'm sure I've said both of those at some point—awful stuff.

The other inane thing people say is, 'Aw, what a great time to score!' I always think, 'Is there ever a bad time?' These inanities are just something to say—they don't actually mean anything.

Funnily enough, I was never particularly comfortable with public speaking prior to becoming a pundit. I'm still not, because I don't do a lot of it. But when I think about it, it's a different discipline anyway. When you're making a speech in public, you are *creating* content. When you're broadcasting, you're reacting to what you're seeing. There's a big difference. Obviously, there's a certain amount of preparation that you should do before you go on TV—there's information you should know in advance: who's playing well; who's not; what's the form of the teams; who's injured; how long's someone been injured; who's just coming back.

You know all that, so what can go wrong? You know the game itself inside out, so you just sit there and react. In my mind it's like me sitting on the couch, watching the game with you. At halftime, before you go and make a cup of tea you go, 'Hey Michael, what was that all about? Why did they do this?'

And I try to answer, in an entertaining, succinct way.

One of the things that irritates me most as a viewer when I watch other sports coverage is when people talk on and on for the sake of filling time. They think that a long explanation or anecdote is good. It's not. You've got to be succinct. To the point, concise … unlike me rabbiting on now. I prefer to approach commentary in a similar way to the late, great Richie Benaud. He was never afraid of silence; he let the pictures tell the story—so much so that sometimes you wondered if he was actually still in the commentary position. Restraint is a fantastic skill to have as a commentator or analyst and I'm always conscious of using it wherever possible.

Obviously I had to learn to alter the depth of my analysis to suit the audience. If it's, say, the Reds versus the Waratahs at 8.30am on a Saturday morning, the people who are watching are probably pretty interested in rugby and know what's going on, to a certain degree. So in that situation I might be a little more technical or detailed in my observations, or conversely might let the pictures speak for themselves.

But if it's the Rugby World Cup on free-to-air television at 7.30pm on a Saturday night, you're going to get viewers who may not know a lot about rugby and you've got to explain the basics a bit more. But not in a condescending way. Often it's the presenter's job to guide the analysis. To prompt the pundits a little. A skilled presenter might ask:

'What do you *mean* when you say he was doing that, Michael?'

'Why was that good?'

'Why was that bad?'

I then have to react to what we're all seeing and give my interpretation of it. My research has been long done, and I talk about what I see, drawing on the information I've uncovered in my preparation. I like doing that.

Q and As at functions are not unlike TV broadcasting; I always really enjoy them. You've got a panel of experts and an audience firing off questions, most of which you've heard many times before. But coming up with interesting answers is the challenge in front of you.

'Who's your toughest opponent?'

'Well, mate, I played top-level rugby for sixteen years ... I could name fifteen,' is what you think. But in reality you've got to make your response to a predictable question entertaining. I usually try to turn it around with a couple of anecdotes, something a bit light-hearted. It's better than trotting out the usual suspects in a dreary list. That's too dry. Too predictable. At every one of those Q and As I do, I know I'll be asked the following questions, though of course there are always some from left field too. But these are the regulars, to which I try to provide interesting answers.

'Who's the best player you've ever played against?'

'Who's the best player you've ever played with?'

And to take the second one, you think to yourself: 'Well, there's John Eales and there's Timmy Horan for starters. You can't compare them. They are different players playing different positions with different sets of skills. Would I have them both in my team? Yes! But you can't say one's better than the other.'

But you have to answer. So you tell a story about Ealesy, a story about Timmy, and a story about Philippe Sella or some other great player you've played with.

Or Campo. I always have a story about him, because people ask me about him every single time.

'What's Campo like?'

And I can't just stand there and say something brief like, 'He's a prick', or 'He's a nice guy.' I've got to say something that gives the people an idea of what he's really like.

While I'm on the subject, I should say that Campo and I always had a good working relationship. I don't usually get the opportunity to go into it in any depth. But because he's one of these guys who always divides opinions, people continue to ask me about him.

In our playing years I got on pretty well with him, particularly early on. Although he's about a year older than me, we played under-21s together. We crossed over into the Australian team together too. Without being what you'd call close, we got on all right. Then, as we got older, we played Sevens together; we roomed together. Not all the time, but whenever we did he was always fine.

As far as his rugby playing was concerned, I'd always have Campo in my team. Whenever I was calling moves of any kind, the first thought that came into my head was always, 'How do I get Campo involved in this move?' Funnily enough, a lot of the time his role was as a decoy. We'd use him, our primary weapon, as a runner, to draw defensive cover away from other players. Most of the time he'd end up on the end of the move anyway, because he was a brilliant, supremely gifted player. Also, back in the amateur days, Campo probably prepared better than anybody. He was in the gym a lot more than anyone else and that was on his own time. In some respects he was way ahead of his time.

He lives in South Africa nowadays. I don't see him very often in person. But every now and then we'll drop each other a note and it's always very friendly. If he came to London and we saw each other at a function, we'd sit and have a chat—no problem at all. I saw him in Hong Kong for the Sevens last year and he was in great form: lots of chat, a great mood. The year before, he wasn't. He wasn't enjoying himself and just wanted to leave. We've all felt like that at some point. That said, when I saw him in Australia in 2014 for the Grand Slam Tour reunion, he was in great form once more.

Like most people, me included, it depends when you catch him. I sometimes have to remind myself, at speaking events or Q and As, how important it can be to people to meet you, talk to you for a minute, get a picture or have something signed.

I was at a Saracens dinner event recently, and by the end I was pretty tired and ready to go home. Just as I was leaving a couple of guys grabbed my arm and said, 'Mate, can you sign this before you go?' They were a bit drunk and then some mates of theirs came along too for a photograph. I said, a little grudgingly, 'All right, here you go. Have a good night.' I was impatient and possibly a bit dismissive.

Isabella said to me on the way home, 'Michael, you should have been nicer to those people.' I said, 'I know, but I'm tired and just want to get home.'

But when I thought about it, she was absolutely right. One of these guys probably told his kids the next morning, 'Oh, that Michael Lynagh, he wasn't very nice.' That makes me think, 'I should have been nicer', especially as I was representing Saracens, in a sense, but you just can't be nice to everyone twenty-four hours a day. Sometimes people catch you at the wrong moment. Or grab your arm, a bit drunk. But I do try to remember, when I'm speaking at an event or sitting on a Q and A panel, that the audience has probably paid money to see me talk. The least I can do is sign something or take a picture with them, but I also think it's fair enough to expect them to approach me in a polite way. Courtesy works both ways, after all.

You also have to remember that audiences, if you've done a lot of these events, as I have, will have heard most of your stories before. So you've got to come up with some new ones every once in a while. What really amuses me is when I tell a true story, then, six months later, I go to a dinner and there's the story, *my* story, being told by someone else with English players' names substituted for the real Australian ones. That happens a lot. I've probably done something similar myself!

COMMENTARY WORK SHOULDN'T BE about predictions and guesswork. Of course you might want to say that a particular game is going to be close or that we might expect to see a lot of tries for a number of different reasons. But predicting a score doesn't mean anything. Nor do expressions like, 'I know it's a cliché but if the forwards can win the ball and the backs can use it, that's the key.'

Yeah, we know that. *Everybody* knows that. You've got to try to say *why* one team is going to get on top. If they've got the better pack of forwards, you've got to say *why* those forwards are better. Everybody knows that if the forwards get on top a team has an advantage, but the most important question is always *why*?

Whenever England play Australia, the same old adages are always applied: England have great forwards and will dominate the scrums, but Australia have better backs. Everybody knows that. So you've got to come up with, for example, a way of explaining how Australia might avoid scrums and keep away from a forward-orientated contest. What tactics might help them do that? It's not easy, but you have to come up with ideas.

I might start by saying, 'Australia needs to move these big English forwards around.' But then I'll also need to say how that might be achieved. I might follow up with 'The Australian lineout is okay. So maybe Australia can play position and use the touchline a bit more to avoid giving England ten-metre scrums where they can push us over and get a penalty try.' One other thing I'm always sceptical about is statistics. They don't always tell the story. A team may have most of the possession and be dominating territory but still might be losing the game. The reason? Forwards won't like me saying this, but getting the ball is the easy part. It's the decisions you make when you've got it and how you execute thereafter that really count.

Why and *how* are the two main questions I always pose in analysis. For instance, it's all very well to say that the flyhalf is really important. Of course he is—he's important for every team in every game. You have to ask yourself *how* he's going to do what he's meant to do and come up with an answer. Then, in the preview, you say it.

I always try to think back to what it's like to be sitting on the couch watching the game with a beer.

'Michael, what exactly has happened there?' the presenter might ask me.

Well, everybody can see that such and such passed the ball to that person, but *who* made the try; *who* made the mistake in defence—that's harder for the average viewer to see, so I'd point that out. If the try came off a good move, I'd show

how it created doubt in the minds of the defence and allowed somebody to go through the gap. I wouldn't just say, 'Great run from Joe Smith to go through the gap.' There's always a *reason* that gap appeared there. It might be that the player inside did a decoy run, or the ball carrier held the ball back. Or it might have happened because the defensive guy came out of the line trying to cover another player he thought would get the ball and created the gap. It's my job to point this out and explain how and why it happened.

It's my background as a player that allows me to do this, and it's why former players appear on TV. Why wouldn't Sky or any other broadcaster use people who are familiar with the game inside out? But in addition to that, it's my job to keep up with how things have changed since I was playing. Rules have changed and the game has become much more physical, so while I played at the highest level, I know that the game has evolved and moved on. If I can't share my knowledge as a player with the viewer, and if I can't keep my knowledge up to date, then Sky might as well get my sister on. She can talk a lot. She's funny. Put *her* on TV.

You've also got to try to add something unique, something that only you have insight into.

'Why did this player get upset and give away a penalty?' the presenter might ask me.

I might answer, 'He dropped the ball earlier or got late tackled, and he's trying to make up for the mistake or get rid of some frustration.'

You often see that with goal-kickers. They'll miss a kick at goal and then they'll do something silly because they're trying to make up for it. That's an insight I can share because it happened to *me*. I learned eventually that you have to separate the two roles. Play, and then when a goal kick comes along, move over to that role. If you've got none out of six, don't try to run the ball from everywhere to make up for it. Kicking and general play are separate parts of the game and you must differentiate them. But it's a very hard thing to do because one affects the other.

I remember one time when Queensland was playing Wellington back in the early '90s. I'd missed a lot of kicks at goal, which was quite normal at Wellington because it's always very windy. The old stadium was up on a hill. But I scored two tries and we won the game. I came off and was interviewed.

'Michael, you got two out of seven but you scored two tries and won the game.'

Then came a typical question from an interviewer who didn't know what to ask next.

'How do you feel?'

I thought, 'Mate, how do you *think* I feel?'

Then I thought a bit more about how I could turn this rather dull question around and make it interesting.

'Well, I feel a little bit like a cricketer who dropped a few catches but scored a hundred. It doesn't matter what I did or didn't do. We won the game.'

Just as when I was playing, I always try to be true to myself when I'm doing television analysis. By nature I'm pretty laidback, pretty calm. Never foaming at the mouth. But nowadays, there seems to be an emphasis on people getting out of their chair and trying to take on a personality that just isn't real. I sometimes get a little carried away, but I've got to be true to my personality. If I'm not, people will sense that and say,

'Nah, that's not him.' If I get genuinely excited, though, it's fine to show it—I think that makes good TV.

Equally, I try not to be slow and dull. Monotonous. The viewer will just go and make a cup of tea. I know I would. If someone is animated, enthusiastic and has a good point of view, people tend to be engaged and keep watching.

SEAN FITZPATRICK: Michael is very professional and always very well prepared. Sometimes we have people who turn up for the job not very well prepared. He always expects other people to be the same way he is: he does not suffer fools and you will never get him to do something he doesn't want to do. I like to think we have a very good working relationship. When he came back after his stroke I said to him, 'Whatever you need, just let me know.' He had a few confidence issues. I always try to be aware of his visual limitations and always think before I put my cup down or my glass down somewhere, 'Is this going to be in his way?'

Occasionally we've had guests on the show who I know are struggling. Maybe it's their first time on TV. They're shy; they're nervous—we've all been in a similar situation. You've almost got to jump in—give them some help, keep things moving along. In a break you say something like, 'Mate, that's great what you were saying there', or, 'That's really good. That's the sort of stuff we want.' You have to be encouraging. A lot of analysis goes on behind the scenes. We'll notice incidents that viewers might not see. Sometimes, if there have been four tries in the first half, we won't have the time to show these minor incidents. But if there's time, we can play them back and talk about them. 'This is why this team is doing so well. Look at this guy. He made a tackle down in that corner, got up, ran into support. Look at him shadowing the runner.' You can track him and show the viewers what's happening.

I remember one incident from 2014 in particular. Brodie Retallick—who I think is a great player—was playing for the Chiefs in the Super 15. He made a tackle at one side of the field, then he went into a ruck and then he was the last defender to make a covering tackle in an attempt to prevent a try. A second-row forward. It didn't matter that the try was scored against him.

'Look at his work rate,' I said.

I stopped the footage for a second and highlighted Brodie.

'He makes a tackle there, goes into a ruck, makes a difference there—and then who's this guy making a tackle in the corner? How does he do that? He's a second-row forward! What great commitment and athleticism.'

By tracking and highlighting good rugby in that way, you can explain to the viewers why it's good play and also why Brodie is a great player. People might not notice otherwise. They just see the try in the corner and the tackle that failed to prevent it.

Equally, when I highlight a mistake, it's not a personal thing. I know all the players are trying hard. I've been there. People don't drop balls on purpose. But as a commentator I can say, 'He's having a shocker—it's just one of those days.'

It's just like when I left my house the other day and slipped in the street on a piece of plywood I didn't see. I fell pretty much flat—I got cuts on my hands and was a bit shaken. Then I got drenched when a bus went through a puddle of water beside me.

Then I arrived at the station to find that my train to work was cancelled. Not delayed—*cancelled*.

Anyone watching this would have said, 'Mate, you are having a shocker!' I thought about turning around and going back to bed.

But instead I grudgingly accepted what had happened and thought, 'Surely it can only get better from here?'

I didn't try to start my day like that—it just happened. Rugby, and any kind of sport, is exactly the same. Sometimes, in these situations, the harder you try, the worse things get. You become tense. You make mistakes. The same applies to referees. They're not trying to make bad decisions. They're not intentionally trying to get things wrong.

But sometimes you've got to point these things out—with both referees and players. That's your job, as a pundit. I usually preface any critique with, 'Look, I know what he was trying to do there ...' Then I add, '... and it was probably the right decision for these reasons.' Then I'd say, 'But his execution was poor.' That way I'm not just having a go. I'm seeing what the player had in mind and explaining why it didn't work out.

Of course, if a player makes three or four mistakes in a row, we'll put them together, and if we have time we'll say, 'Kieran Read at number 8—he's a great player. But he's not having a great day today. Look at this ...' We also do the opposite: 'Look at Kieran Read! What a great day he's having. This is why he's one of the best players in the world.' There's got to be balance.

There also needs to be harmony among us pundits. Sean Fitzpatrick is generally in the studio with me. I enjoy Fitzy's company. He likes to stir things up a little—wind me up a bit to get a reaction. He's pretty good at that and that's what he used to do on the field. I'll say, 'The All Blacks get preferential treatment from every referee', or 'Look at McCaw! Let's just look at the replay and you tell me that this is not offside.'

Fitzy just shakes his head. I've got him to agree with me most of the time now.

But then he'll turn it back on me. 'Look at Hooper! He's *always* offside. Come on!'

Having said all that, we have a pretty good time considering we never got on particularly well on the field. He was always really obnoxious on the pitch. Even he wouldn't deny that. It was part of what made him so great. He took every opportunity to wind you up. For example, whenever you were getting up from the ground after a tackle and Fitzy was running past, he'd make a point of standing on your hand. Every single time, his studs would crunch into the back of your hand. Fitzy never missed an opportunity to irritate you and wear you down—that's just how he played the game. He also knew exactly how to get referees onside. He'd give you a clip round the ear as he ran past and if you reacted in any way he'd say: 'Aw, come on, ref! Michael's pretty tense today. You'd better calm him down.'

SEAN FITZPATRICK: We never got on particularly well [on the field], to be honest. We were just a grizzly bunch of bloody forwards who annoyed the hell out of the Aussies. That was always the All Black mentality: look for a chink in the armour and then try to exploit it. I was horrible—a horrible person [on the field]. I think the Aussies were always vulnerable to our antics. I remember Simon Poidevin at the bottom of a ruck, while I'm standing on his head, yelling, 'Fitzpatrick, I'm going to get you!'

I played against Michael all the way back to the under-21s and he was always a class above everyone else. I remember playing him in 1982 or '83—he was at a completely different level. Michael was one of those special cases. Even when I watched him play outside Ella at number 12 on the Grand Slam tour in 1984, he had maturity way beyond his years.

TWENTY-ONE

THE TOUR LIKE NO OTHER

ALTHOUGH I WAS STILL contracted to Sky, I was left out of the team for the 2013 Lions tour to Australia. They wanted a British- and Irish-dominated studio and that, I suppose, made sense. I was disappointed—of course I was—in the same way that I was whenever I was dropped from any team. But you can either go away and moan about it, focusing on the negatives, or you can say, 'I see where they're coming from', and look upon it as an opportunity to do something else. I chose the latter.

There were no hard feelings on my end whatsoever. Nevertheless, I was still very keen to go. It would be great to spend six weeks in Australia watching the tour. Some of the time would be spent in Melbourne, and I thought, 'That would be great—I've hardly ever spent any time there.'

So I was excited to be offered the chance to work with Jim Rosenthal, Scott Gibbs, Jeremy Guscott and Steve Thompson on a panel for OSN Sports, a Dubai-based pay TV network that was also covering the series. On paper it was a great bunch of guys, some of whom I'd worked with before. An agent contacted me: 'Do you fancy it?' and I said, 'Yes, I'd love to do it.' There were no downsides for me whatsoever. I'd cover the action, enjoy great synergy with the other panellists and spend six weeks in Australia. And get paid for doing so. Yes, it was a long time away from home but it seemed to pass quickly and was worth it on a financial level. Not just that, but from an ambassadorial point of view, there were plenty of speaking opportunities for me on the radio, on television and at live events.

The Lions tour is a huge sporting event nowadays, arguably on a par with the Ryder Cup or the Tour de France. The nation, or in this case several nations, stops to watch, even though the sport of rugby union is still a distant fourth in terms of popularity in Australia.

Inevitably, as an Australian who's played in a Lions series, I was often asked during the 2013 tour for my thoughts on that Lions tour to Australia in 1989. That was always a bit of a problem because, as with most matches and series, I just don't remember many of the details. I really have to dig deep to dredge them up. 'What was that game again? What happened *there*? Jeez, I'll really have to give this some thought.'

What most people forget is that 1989 was the first full Lions tour to Australia, so we didn't really have anything to measure it against. In that sense, it was a bit like the 1987 World Cup: there was no precedent. Australia had previously been just a stop-off for the Lions on the way to New Zealand, so we didn't have the same Lions traditions as South Africa and New Zealand, and the concept of the Lions coming for a three-Test tour wasn't something especially important. Also, until that point, and not wishing to sound arrogant, we'd largely beaten the northern hemisphere sides quite comfortably. While we still weren't professional or employing professional methods, I always felt that we were physically better than they were. We were naturally physically fitter.

Why was that? Well, I've often thought about it and I keep coming back to the lifestyle we were able to lead in Australia. When I was a kid, I was outside every afternoon, running around. Playing sport of some kind every day. I was fit. We were all fit. And that wasn't just because we were running more laps of the oval than anyone else. Yes, when we thought of 'fitness', the first idea that came into our heads was, 'Let's go, ten laps of the oval—quick as you can.' But there was a *broader* type of fitness that only a southern hemisphere upbringing could give you: the climate, being outside all the time in the fresh air, surfing every week. It all added up, making us stronger.

I never went to the gym. I hated the gym. But I was training every day in some way: a game of touch down the park, surfing, cricket training, playing tennis on my friend's tennis court. Non-stop activity. But it didn't feel like we were consciously trying to get fit.

We were fit simply because there was always something to keep the body active and the weather was conducive to doing it. I'd come home only when it got dark and get up and do the same thing the next day. I really believe that made a big difference. We were stronger and harder than northern hemisphere teams then as a result. So when things got tough in the last fifteen minutes of games, we had the edge because of our upbringing. That was the theory. The same applies to New Zealanders and South Africans; we share that same inherent toughness, although I've often thought that the inability to tap into a vein of farming stock has been where Australia has been at a disadvantage compared with the All Blacks and the Springboks. Most Australian players have come from city backgrounds.

The gap has closed now, obviously. Now every team has indoor facilities and specialised nutrition and training and it makes no difference where you grow up. But back in the amateur days there was a significant gulf in fitness between teams from the northern and southern hemispheres.

Having now spent quite some time living in the northern hemisphere, I know that it gets dark at 3.30pm in winter. If I was a kid, the last thing I'd want to do is go outside and play sport, although my own kids manage it fine nowadays, probably because they've known nothing else. Even when I was playing for Saracens as a professional, I used to say to myself, 'If I'd grown up here, I would not have become a rugby player.' You adjust, but it's just not pleasant. Instead of being outside in January, I'd rather be at home in front of the fire with the paper and a glass of red wine.

So when the Lions came over to Australia in 1989, I thought, 'Well, it's just another northern hemisphere team and we've beaten all of them already.' It might sound cocky, but that was really how it seemed. We thought, 'We'll give them a bit of a touch-up as well.' We felt that we had each of these countries' measure.

Of course, they'd beaten us reasonably regularly prior to when I started playing. But after 1984, apart from a defeat against England at Twickenham in 1988 in Will Carling's first game as captain, we'd had pretty much constant victory over all of the countries that make up the Lions. And there were even a few valid excuses for our Twickenham loss. Why would this be any different? I felt no more threatened than I might have felt if it was England or Wales on tour.

Despite the way I felt, everybody kept saying, 'But it's the Lions' first tour ...' as if it was a big deal.

It didn't matter. The way I approached it was still, 'Okay, here's another job to be done.' That was my way of focusing on any match, no matter who the opposition was. When I think about it now, though, I would say that I misjudged the Lions tour in 1989. Perhaps that's only because the Lions tour is such a huge deal nowadays and there *is* a tradition in Australia. Back then I was a little naive about it.

As it turned out, it was an exciting three-match series with a famous moment in the third match that still lives on today. That third Test match, though ... what a shocker that turned into.

As I recall, ten minutes from the end, Rob Andrew had an attempt at drop goal that went out to the right. I was standing on the twenty-two; we were ahead at the time. We were reasonably in control; they were having occasional shots at drop goal; there wasn't much more in their arsenal. We were holding them. Frustrating them. Our forwards were immense. I thought, 'Okay, we've got this.'

To be completely fair to Campo, he hadn't had a lot of ball that day. It had been a tight game, not particularly expansive, and Campo was stuck out there on his left wing. He didn't like that. His excuse for what happened next was, 'Well, I hadn't had a lot of ball so I had to use every opportunity.' So he gathered Rob Andrew's missed drop goal in the dead ball area, and instead of just touching it down as he should have and giving us a twenty-two drop-out, he tried to run it out. To be fair to him, if he'd gone on his own he probably would have gained a lot of ground. Instead, he flipped this pass to Greg Martin while they were both still on the goal line. The decision itself wasn't a bad one, on reflection. It was two on one with the Lions' wing Ieuan Evans, and in rugby language two on one usually means 'take it on'. Just not behind your own try line.

Also, his execution let him down. It wasn't a great pass. Although he'd throw a few very important passes later in his career, Campo wasn't really known for his passing. It was short and a little behind Greg. Secondly, Greg wasn't expecting it. He must have thought, 'Why on earth are you passing to me *here*?' Ieuan Evans, who simultaneously must have been thinking, 'It's Christmas!' got in the middle of it and just fell on the ball.

It was a calamity and, worse than that, it was totally unnecessary. I just dropped to my knees on the twenty-two and thought, 'Oh God, what's he done? After all this work …'

I don't know what the forwards felt—they work a lot harder than we do, putting themselves physically on the line all day, just so we can look good. But we all had to run back behind the goal line and wait for the conversion. It wasn't the way you expect to lose a game.

To lose a *series*.

What was said to Campo in the dressing room afterwards? Not much. It was pretty stony, I can tell you. But it was only really stony because we'd lost—and it was normally pretty quiet when we lost anyway. But this was just such a silly way to lose. It doubled the disappointment.

We all went to the after-match reception and, of course, the Lions were on fire, buying Campo champagne, all having a great time—'We've beaten the Aussies on their own patch, lads!'

Legend has it that Campo went home early from the reception and got pulled over by the police as he was driving to his place in Bondi—speeding, sirens, the whole palaver. He winds down the window and the policeman comes over. Then Campo apparently says, 'Mate, I've had a really crap day but, yeah, I was probably speeding. I just want to go home.' As the policeman's writing out the ticket, he goes, 'Yeah, I know. I was there. I watched you, you prick.'

On reflection, the second Test was one that we should have won as well. The first Test we had won easily, 31–12 in Sydney. It wasn't really much of a contest. The Lions were just finding their range and ours—'What have you got?'

For the second Test up in Brisbane the Lions had a specific method. It was, 'Let's target their halfback.' They figured that they couldn't stop guys like Campo and me running the game, so they thought, 'Okay, how do we stop the ball getting to them? Let's cut off the supply.'

So they decided to upset our captain, Nick, by basically making the game one long physical fight. It worked. Nick was a very fair player who always played within the rules, but if he was confronted he was not the kind of guy who would lie down. Right from the first scrum when Robert Jones stood on his foot, it was on.

Once they'd upset Nick, they started kicking at Campo, kicking behind him, putting pressure on him all the time. The Lions were just a different team from the first Test. Both in personnel and, more importantly, the way they came out. They were very aggressive towards us. Nasty.

Until that point, we had prided ourselves on our ability to not give away penalties. We were not a dirty team. We were tough but never undisciplined, but they came out wanting to physically fight us, and that really put us off our game. I think they sensed that we were a little bit soft when it came to an all-out fistfight; it wasn't our nature to do that kind of stuff.

I was targeted too, as I was in every game I played. Years later, when Jonny Wilkinson came on the scene, people said, 'Aw, they're targeting Jonny. Running down his channel. With his sore shoulder', as if it was something new.

I used to think to myself, 'Show me a flyhalf in the history of the game who hasn't been targeted!' It's like targeting the quarterback in American football. It's the logical place to start. He's the conductor. Take him out and the orchestra can't play. Equally, the flyhalf is the playmaker—of course he's going to get targeted.

In the first Test, they couldn't really get anywhere near me. The guys were running at me, trying to get to me, but I didn't mind that because it created more space for the people around me. Any time people ran really hard at me when I had the ball, I liked it. They were so intent on hitting me that I could easily move the ball on. I'd think, 'Okay, that takes *you* out of the game.'

Dirty play could be painful. If I was tackled late, that would hurt. But it would also mean a penalty, and I'd say, 'Thanks very much mate, that was good.' And add three points to our score, or gain territory or some kind of an advantage. That just riled opponents even more. Sometimes, as I was lining up the kick from the penalty they'd just given away, someone might have a chirp at me during my run-up—'I've seen you miss this one before, mate.' That stuff you have to just block out. Backchat was all part of the game. There's probably less of it nowadays because the players all know each other so well. The game was certainly a lot dirtier in my time. And even dirtier *before* my time. Today there are cameras everywhere and the referees and linesmen are trained professionals. Also, if you get caught nowadays, you're out for a few games and games equal money in today's world. It's a different environment altogether.

Now, of course, the Lions tour is a huge tradition in Australia. So much so that if it wasn't for the 2013 Lions tour, the Australian Rugby Union would be pretty close to the financial wall now. They don't have much money. The situation really isn't good. Rugby union is still a minority sport in Australia. I'd love to find a way to change that but I can't help thinking that it will be very difficult. Let's just hope that the Lions' tradition of touring Australia and everywhere else continues; it's a great event to be involved with, as a player or a pundit.

While I was out in Australia covering the Lions, I gave a number of speeches and sat on some Q and A panels. Dad and a few friends whom I hadn't seen for a while came to a couple of them in Brisbane, and it was great to have them there. After one of them Dad said to me, 'That was great. You really stood out up there.' I liked getting that affirmation from him. At another one, where I knew I hadn't done so well, he said, 'The MC wasn't great, was he?'

To be fair, the format had been awkward. I'd wanted to speak on my own but the guy wouldn't let me. Instead, he

TWENTY-TWO
MUCH MORE TO DO

IT'S 2015, THREE YEARS down the road from the stroke. Sometimes it feels as if it was years ago—another lifetime. Other times it seems like it happened last week. Sometimes I feel that I'd like to put the whole series of events behind me and forget it happened, but other times I want to hold on to what happened always. Like it or not, the stroke is part of me now—the person I now am has been significantly influenced by those events of April 2012. I've had the stroke experience, along with thousands of others in my life. They all make me the person I now am. I can only take the good with the bad and the former still vastly outweighs the latter.

Stroke has taught me a lot about certain aspects of myself, and, as someone who has always been hungry for information, that's no bad thing. I'm not somebody who can sit back and say, 'Okay, this is where I am and it's not going to get better.' I always want to improve my situation and my stroke recovery has been a daily mission to achieve that. Even if I hadn't had the stroke, I'd still be trying to improve my situation. That never stops for me.

I still wake up in the morning sometimes and think, 'You know what, my eyesight might be a bit better.' Maybe it is; maybe I'm just imagining it is. Either way, it doesn't matter. It's the hope and the positivity that go into thinking it might improve that are important.

Obviously, I still can't drive and that's an ongoing problem. I say 'still', because I genuinely believe that I will be able to one day. I have occasional eye examinations to check my peripheral vision. They put me in a chair looking at a board onto which they flash a series of dots and they ask me to pull a trigger when I see them. What you have to remember is that my eyes, in strict terms, are as good as they were before the stroke. It's the message that's sent to my brain that has been damaged by the stroke, not the eyes themselves. *That's* what dictates what I actually see.

There's a test that you need to pass before you can resume driving, but if you fail it, you can't sit it again unless you can prove beyond doubt that your vision has improved. I'm getting close to the point where I think I might be able to sit the test.

The only other symptom I have remaining from the stroke is a strange sensation of heat on the lower part of my left leg. It can be quite painful and even wakes me up at night sometimes. In my occasional communications with Rob Henderson, and at the routine follow-up appointments I attend with the specialists in London who now have my file, I've asked what this could be. Nobody has a definitive answer. The brain is a complex organ, even in people who've never had a stroke. Sometimes the body will experience pain or a sensation and it's hard to trace the cause.

In my case, where I've had a major brain injury and will always, even in a small way, be recovering from it, the cause of the burning sensation is almost impossible to figure out. It might be some kind of cross-lateral manifestation from one of the areas of damage in the right side of my brain. It might just as easily be nothing to do with that. It's irritating, but in the scheme of things it really isn't important. I'm just the kind of guy who likes to know what's going on in his body. My mind, as I've noted, is never very quiet.

Mortality is something that I wrestled with for quite some time. I'm trying to remember if I ever did prior to the stroke and I don't think I ever gave it more than a 'Well, I'm getting a bit older' type of thought. I'm not sure if anyone in their forties does unless they're suddenly faced with it when they least expect it. I certainly don't lie in bed at night thinking, 'What if I have another stroke?'—let's put it that way. I'm sure Isabella and the kids still worry about me, but there's part of me that thinks, perhaps naively, 'I survived this, I can do anything.'

That doesn't mean that I do reckless things, not at all. But it does mean that I can approach life with a degree of comfort, knowing that I can fight for my life, not just for a win on the rugby field. The mentality is the same, however: you pull yourself out of danger by setting small, achievable goals, and in the end you'll get the outcome that you've set your mind to. You have to think like that, or else what's the point in living.

Thankfully, the specialists reckon that my chances of having another stroke are no higher than for any normal person of my age and fitness. I assumed I'd be more susceptible, simply because I'd had one already. That's not the case. So I can live, work and enjoy life with very few limitations on what I can and can't do. I'm so lucky in that respect. All those events that went through my head in hospital: my sons going to university, weddings, first cars—their whole lives. It was the thought of not being there that kept me going, and I'm elated to have all of that in front of me. I know how things could have turned out, because I've seen people who've been far less fortunate than me. And, of course, a significant number of stroke victims don't survive at all.

Most significantly, the stroke has put my rugby career in perspective. While there were several parallels in terms of how I approached each discipline, I don't seriously compare recovering from stroke with playing rugby. Rugby is a game, a great game with fabulous traditions. I'm lucky enough to be held in pretty good regard by most people who know anything about the game. The level of support I received and still receive is tremendous. The stroke was about surviving and being around to continue the fifty-plus year journey I've been on. It's that simple.

I've been lucky enough to have enjoyed a good life so far, in every respect. Great marriage, fantastic kids, played sport for my country, won a World Cup, got to travel and meet wonderful people … and yes, I've survived a stroke too. All these things combine to make me what I am and make me content. But me having survived a stroke will not dictate or influence my life from now on. It was an obstacle—a big one, but it's just part of the whole picture. I'm certainly not sitting back in my rocking chair with my slippers on saying, 'Ah, life's winding down now.' There's still a lot of life to live—watching my kids grow up—and thank goodness I can do that. Remember, there was that time where I was thinking that they'd be okay without me. Now though, I've got a lot of living still to do. I've got an eight-year-old son so I've got to be on my toes for the next few years!

WHAT IS A STROKE?

- A stroke is a medical emergency.
- A stroke is the way we describe the blood supply to the brain being suddenly cut off.
- This can happen in two ways: Blood can stop moving through the artery when it gets blocked by a clot or when an artery bursts.
- Brain cells can quickly die without the oxygen that the blood supplies.
- This is why it is so important to get to hospital immediately if you think you are having a stroke because it is possible there may be some cells that can survive if you are treated quickly.

RECOGNISING SIGNS OF STROKE

The FAST test is an easy way to remember and recognise the signs of stroke.

Stroke is **always** a medical emergency. Even if the symptoms don't cause pain or go away quickly – call 000 immediately. The longer a stroke remains untreated, the greater the chance of stroke related brain damage. Emergency medical treatment soon after stroke symptoms begin improves the chances of survival and successful rehabilitation.

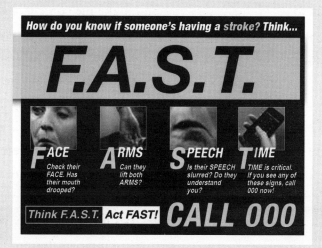

Know your risk factors and lower your risk

Risk factor	How it affects your risk of stroke	Lifestyle changes to lower your risk	Key message
High blood pressure	Causes damage to blood vessel walls eventually leading to a stroke. High blood pressure is one of the most important risk factors for stroke.	• Be smoke free. • Maintain a healthy lifestyle. • Reduce salt intake. • Limit alcohol intake. • Your doctor may prescribe medication.	Know your blood pressure and check it regularly.
Smoking	Increases blood pressure and reduces oxygen in the blood.	Stop smoking.	Be smoke free.
High blood cholesterol	Contributes to blood vessel disease often leading to a stroke.	• Maintain a healthy lifestyle. • Choose foods low in saturated fat. • Your doctor may prescribe medication.	Check your blood cholesterol level.
Diabetes	Can cause damage to the circulatory system and can increase risk of stroke.	• Maintain a healthy body weight. • Keep blood pressure and blood cholesterol levels down.	Talk to your doctor about keeping diabetes under control.
Being overweight	High body fat can contribute to high blood pressure, cholesterol and lead to heart disease, type 2 diabetes and stroke.	• Maintain a healthy body weight. • Be physically active.	Talk to your doctor, a dietitian or a nutritionist for help. Be active everyday.
Poor diet and inactivity	Can contribute to high cholesterol, high blood pressure and lead to obesity increasing risk of stroke.	• Maintain a healthy body weight. • Be physically active. • Eat foods that are good for you.	Talk to your doctor, a dietitian or a nutritionist for help. Be active everyday.
Excessive alcohol	Can raise blood pressure and increase your risk of stroke.	Stay within recommended limits (no more than 2 drinks per day).	Limit your alcohol intake.
Atrial Fibrillation (AF)	You are more at risk of stroke if you have an irregular pulse due to atrial fibrillation.	Follow general advice to lower risk factors.	If you experience symptoms such as palpitations, weakness, faintness or breathlessness, see your doctor for diagnosis or treatment.

The more risk factors you have, the higher your chances of having a stroke. Talk to your doctor about calculating your overall risk of stroke and heart attack.

REDUCING YOUR RISK OF STROKE

There are **6 steps** people can take to reduce the risk and the danger of stroke. These are:

1. Know your personal risk factors: high blood pressure, diabetes and high blood cholesterol – Know your numbers.
2. Be physically active and exercise regularly.
3. Avoid obesity by keeping to a healthy diet.
4. Limit alcohol consumption.
5. Avoid cigarette smoke. If you smoke, seek help to stop now.
6. Learn to recognise the warning signs of a stroke and act FAST.

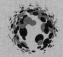

strokefoundation

Information courtesy of the National Stroke Foundation
Level 7, 461 Bourke Street
Melbourne VIC 3000
Phone: 03 9670 1000
Email: admin@strokefoundation.com.au
We have offices in Brisbane, Canberra, Sydney, Hobart and Perth.

StrokeLine 1800 787 653
www.facebook.com/strokefoundation
@strokefdn
www.strokefoundation.com.au

UK residents, please contact the UK Stroke Association
240 City Road, London, EC1V 2PR
Phone: 020 7566 0300
Fax: 020 7490 2686
Textphone: 18001 0303 3033 100
www.stroke.org.uk
Stroke Helpline: 0303 303 3100.
The helpline is open Monday to Friday, 9am to 5pm.

ACKNOWLEDGMENTS

THERE ARE SO MANY people to thank regarding this project and in my life in general.

To all the people in the rugby world I have played with and against, who have coached and cajoled me and in some way contributed to my wonderful rugby life. Thank you. It has been an extraordinary journey—one to which I owe everything. Thanks too to those of you who were called upon to contribute interviews and to Alan Jones for his wonderful foreword.

To Dr. Robert Henderson, Dr. Craig Winter, their wonderful team and the incredible staff in the intensive care unit at the Royal Brisbane and Women's hospital—you are amazing. You deal with adversity and extreme stress everyday with care, calmness and professionalism beyond what can be reasonably expected.

To all the people at HarperCollins both in Australia and the UK —thank you for your belief in this project. My friends at Essentially who put together the deal for me— many thanks to you too.

A huge debt of gratitude to Mark Eglinton who helped me put this story together. We had not previously met and we originally connected via social media, several months after my stroke, where we discussed the idea of doing a book. Although he was not from a rugby journalism background, what he brought from other areas of life, in combination with his understanding of the game, was very appealing. He convinced me—by writing a sample based on one of our first conversations—that people *would actually* be interested in my story. Quite simply, he was able to capture the story and my personality very well. Mark has helped every step of the way and has moulded our many conversations into what you now have in your hands. This book would not have happened without his enthusiasm, passion and interest in it. It has been a pleasure working with him and I feel we have become good friends. Thank you, Mark, you have been magnificent. Thanks also must go to Mark's wife, Linda, for putting up with her husband speaking to me at all hours of the day.